The guide to
OPTIMIZING RECOVERY
After Prostate
Cancer Surgery

The guide to
OPTIMIZING RECOVERY
After Prostate
Cancer Surgery

2nd Edition

SAMANTHA HUGHES, MScPT

Registered Physiotherapist
and Pelvic Health
Educator

Edited by
Claude Cartelier

Design by
Adriana Melo

Ilustrations by
Adriano Renzi

Reviewer
Penny Wilson

ISBN: 978-1-9990680-2-8

Note from the author:
Although every effort has been made to ensure that the information presented in this book is correct, the author cannot be held responsible for any injuries that may arise.

🌐 www.samhughes.ca

@ sam@samhughes.ca

📷 @samhughesphysiotherapy

British Columbia | Canada
2024

Acknowledgements

I would like to thank Pat Lieblich from B.C. Women's Health Centre for allowing me to use her handouts, and Penny Wilson for her words of encouragement.

I would also like to thank Dr. Samarasekera and Dr. Kwan for their contributions to this book and for supporting me in this endeavour.

Lastly, I would like to thank my editor Claude Cartelier for helping me make this book user friendly and for all his great suggestions and remarks.

This book is dedicated to my grandfather Dr. Orlando Baiocchi, who was one of the pioneers in Brazilian Cervical Cancer Research and who died of prostate cancer in 1997.

Table of Contents

Prostate cancer is the 2nd most common form of cancer in men worldwide (1), with increasing incidence rates - especially in North America, New Zealand and northern Europe (2). Medical advancements in early detection and treatment have been resulting in an increasing rate of prostate cancer survivors (3). Unfortunately, most prostate cancer treatments – including radical prostatectomy, radiation and hormonal therapy – have side effects which can immensely impact men's emotional state and overall quality of life.

Radical prostatectomy surgery is one of the main causes for urinary incontinence (4) and erectile dysfunction in men. Side effects such as these can greatly affect men and their loved ones, that's why receiving the right education at the right time can help in the recovery process. Unfortunately there seems to be a lack of or conflicting information on how to manage prostate surgery side effects. Uncertainty contributes to stress and anxiety, which can affect the overall healing process.

This book was developed to cover the need for more information on how to best manage the side effects of prostate surgery. It can be used as a guide for men that elected to have surgery and want to learn more about the recovery process. It summarizes the surgery, bladder physiology, pelvic floor muscle training, and behavioural changes to improve urinary incontinence, and other possible side effects. The information herein has been carefully collected from clinical expertise and research, and has been written in an easy-to-read format with pertinent illustrations.

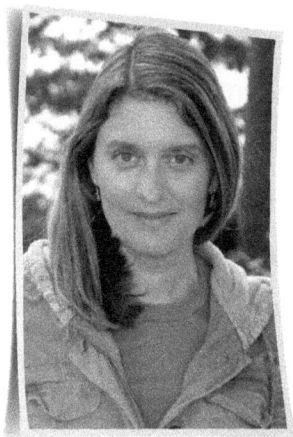
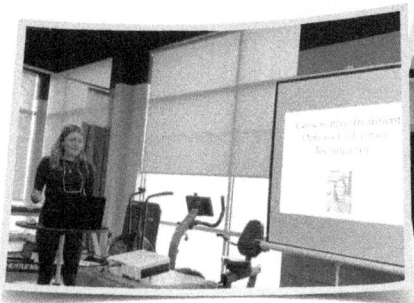
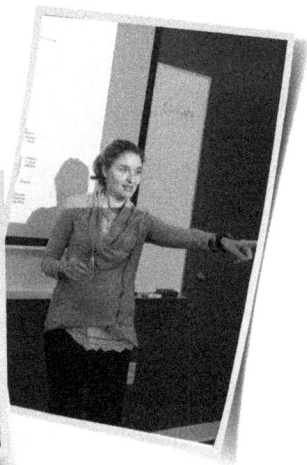
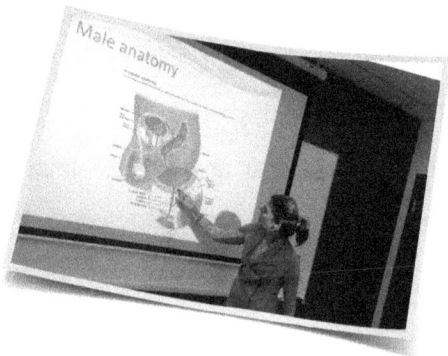

The Author

Samantha Hughes is a licensed physical therapist working in British Columbia, Canada. She has a Masters degree from the University of Alberta, Canada, and extensive advanced certification in women's, men's, and pelvic floor health. She has been the spokesperson for various prostate support groups and conferences. After conducting research in the area of incontinence post-prostatectomy, Samantha Hughes implemented the prostatectomy physical therapy program at the Jim Pattison Outpatient Clinic, one of British Columbia's largest public bladder clinics. She is an advocate for empowering clients with knowledge and education, simplifying complicated information to be easily understood by the public. She is constantly creating opportunities to educate the public and health professionals about pelvic floor physical therapy, regularly giving public presentations and speaking at medical meetings. She has created various study groups among her peers and has provided mentorship to new pelvic floor physical therapists. Samantha Hughes is well-respected by the medical community and thrives to provide the best possible care.

Having extensively treated incontinent men post-radical prostatectomy, Samantha Hughes found that the lack of education was impacting men's outcome post-surgery. The aim of this book is to compile relevant information to help improve knowledge regarding prostate cancer surgery recovery.

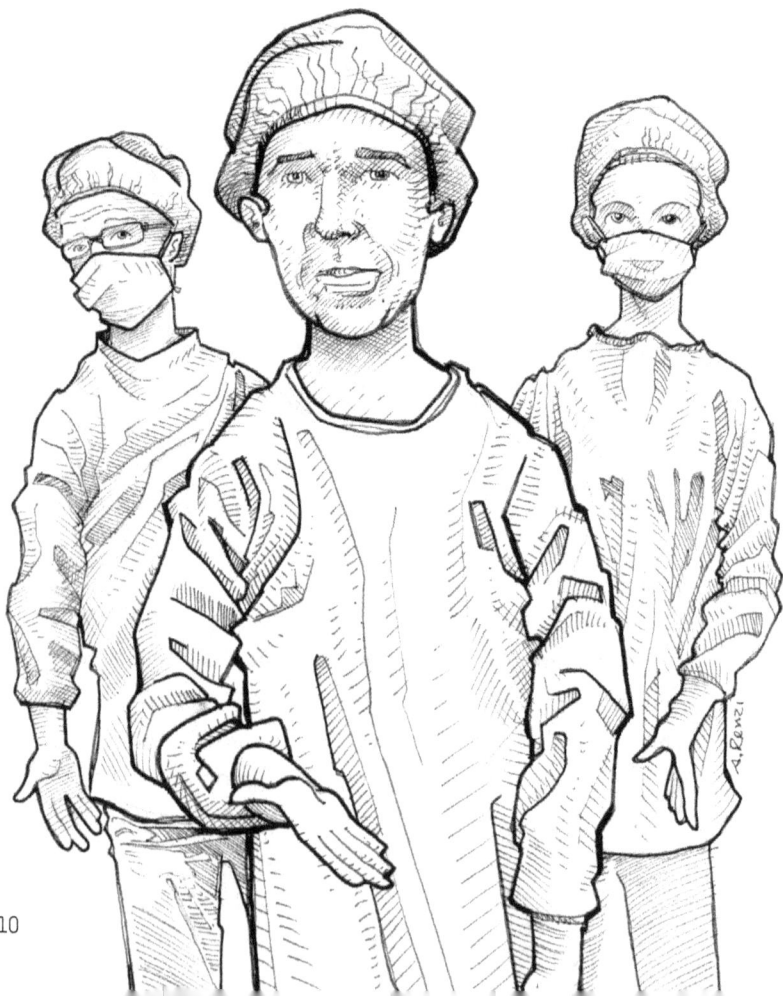

Chapter 1

Prostatectomy Surgery

Radical Prostatectomy surgery (removal of the entire prostate) is performed to treat localized prostate cancer, and has the best incidence of survival rate of all prostate cancer treatments (5). There are different types of radical prostatectomy procedures: laparoscopic, robotic, retropubic, and nerve sparing. Usually, the type of procedure is dependent on the surgeon's expertise and/or preference.

During a radical prostatectomy, the surgeon's main objective is to remove the cancer with clear surgical margins. Occasionally, nerve bundles and adjacent glands are also removed to lessen the chances of the cancer spreading.

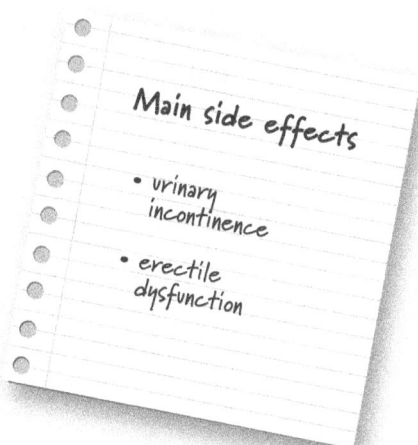

Main side effects

- urinary incontinence
- erectile dysfunction

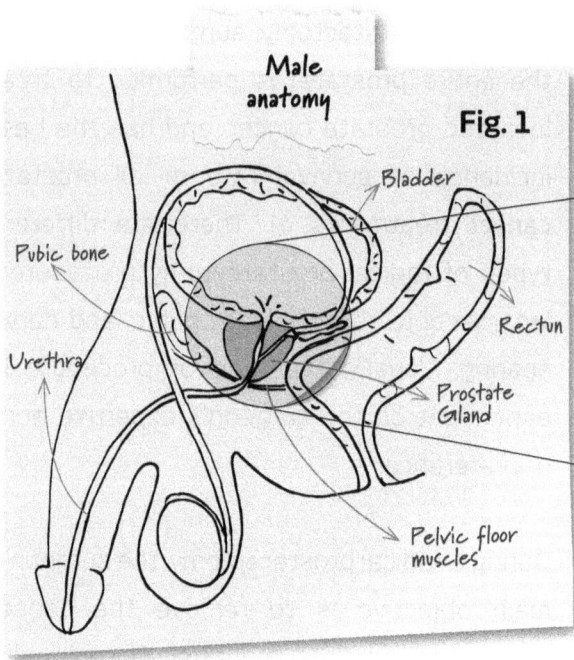

Male anatomy

Fig. 1

Bladder

Pubic bone

Rectum

Urethra

Prostate Gland

Pelvic floor muscles

With any surgery there are potential side effects. One of the most common side effects of radical prostatectomy surgery is urinary incontinence. Anatomical changes after surgery can contribute to urinary incontinence. When the prostate and internal sphincter are removed a space is created and the bladder descends. Damage to the

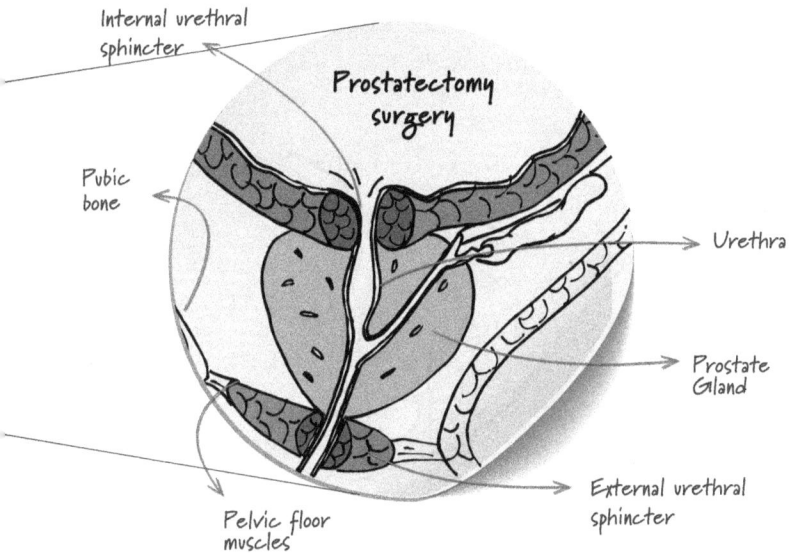

Internal urethral sphincter

Prostatectomy surgery

Pubic bone

Urethra

Prostate Gland

Pelvic floor muscles

External urethral sphincter

external urethral sphincter muscles can also occur and contribute to urine leakage **(Fig. 1)**. The internal and external urethral sphincters are valves that control urinary leakage. When these valves are damaged or removed, it will result in less urinary control. (More information on bladder physiology and urinary control is explained in Chapter 2).

Fig. 2

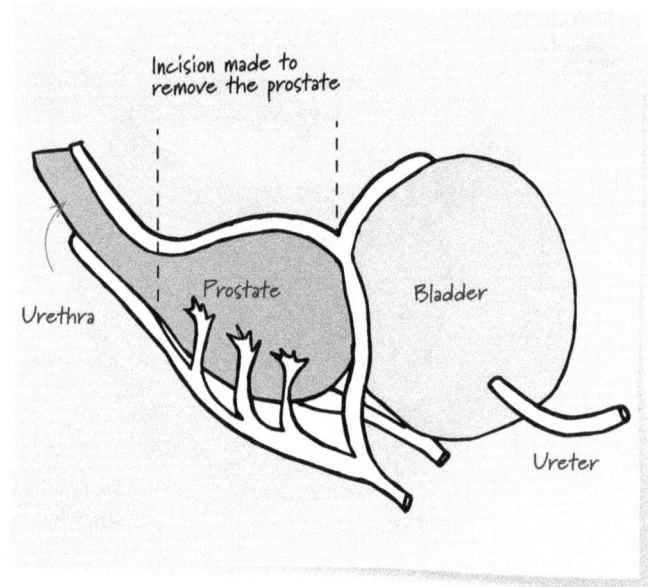

Incision made to remove the prostate

Prostate

Urethra

Bladder

Ureter

The urethra is the tube that extends from the bladder, through the prostate gland all the way down the penis, ending at the tip (external orifice). When radical prostatectomy surgery is performed, removal of the prostate gland (and part of the internal urethral sphincter) is followed by the re-attachment of the urethra to the bladder. A catheter is then inserted to maintain the bladder opening and allow urine drainage. The catheter stays inserted for about 2 weeks after the surgery for healing

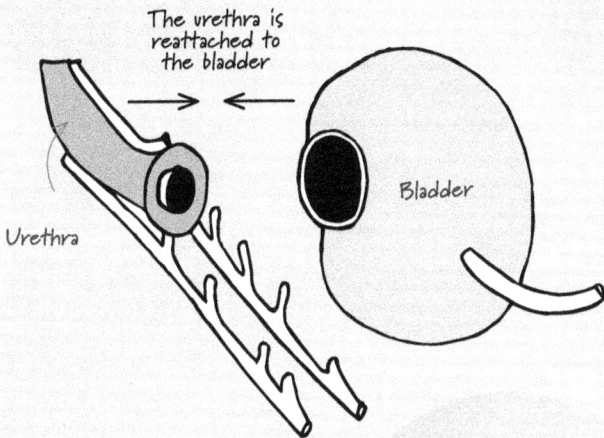

The urethra is reattached to the bladder

Urethra

Bladder

There are different types of radical prostatectomy procedures: laparoscopic, robotic, retropubic, and nerve sparing.

to occur around the opening without blocking urine passage. Once the catheter is removed, urination should occur without difficulties **(Fig. 2)**. The bladder then descends to accommodate for the space left from removal of the prostate gland. A nerve-sparing procedure may enable men to achieve spontaneous erections in the future.

Notes

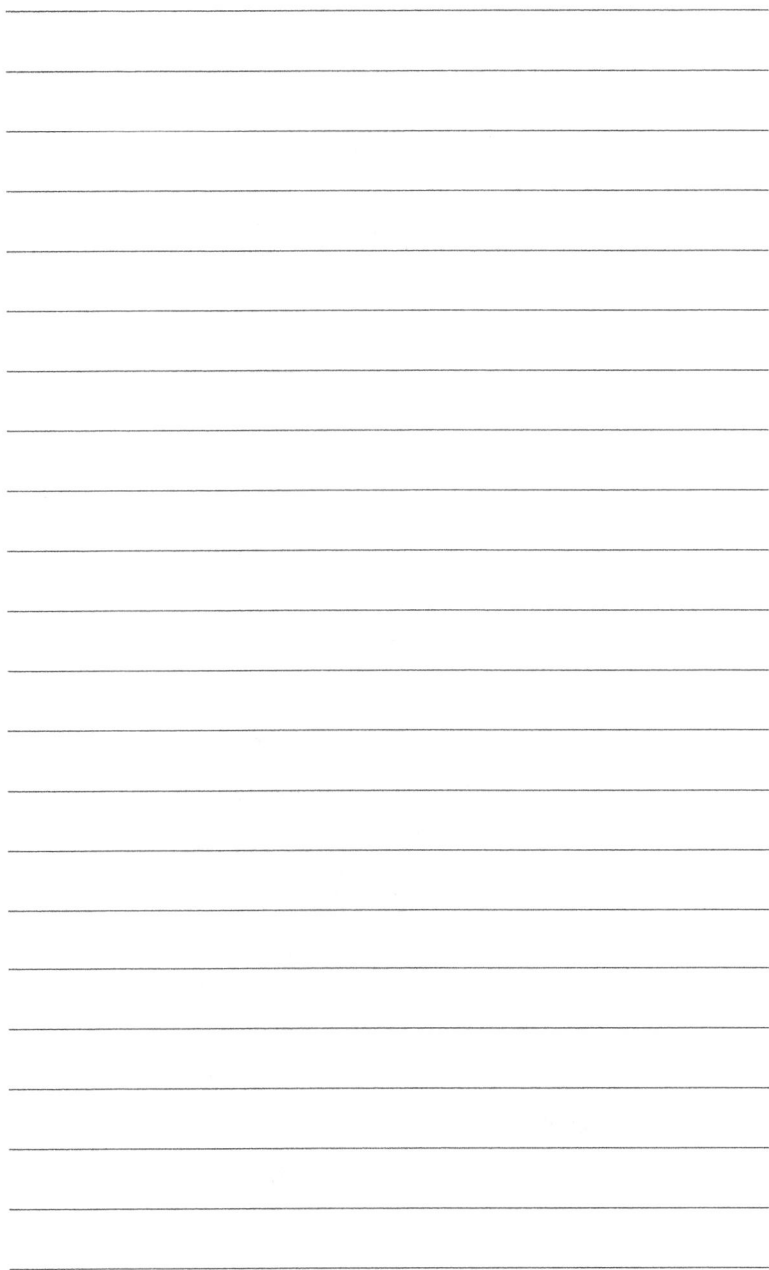

Chapter 2
Urinary Mechanism and Bladder Physiology

To understand bladder recovery it is important to understand bladder and sphincter physiology and function **(Fig. 3)**.

The bladder is a hollow organ whose main function is to store urine prior to urination. Urine is produced in the kidneys and transported to the urinary bladder to be stored. Storage is possible mostly due to the internal and external urethral sphincters. These sphincters close the urethra in two main separate locations to allow urine to be stored in the bladder. The internal urethral sphincter is involuntary, whereas the external urethral sphincter has voluntary control.

When the bladder is half full, information is automatically sent from the bladder to nerves in the sacrum and back, contracting the bladder and relaxing the internal urethral sphincter. This process is called the micturition reflex. To avoid involuntary urination, the external urethral sphincter - controlled by higher centers in the brain - contracts and the bladder then relaxes until the person chooses an appropriate time to urinate.

Fig. 3

Bladder physiology
(full and empty)

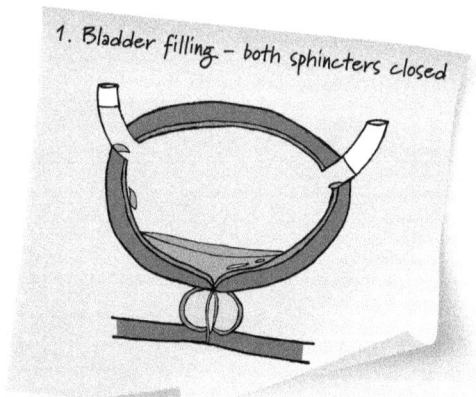

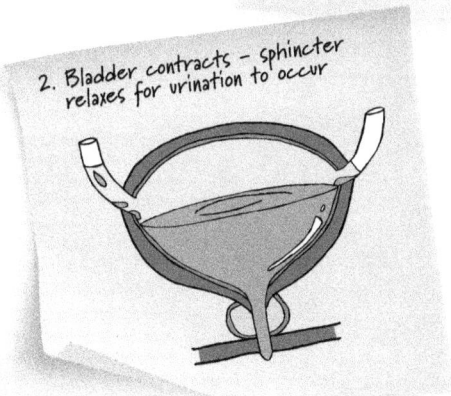

1. Bladder filling – both sphincters closed

2. Bladder contracts – sphincter relaxes for urination to occur

Notes

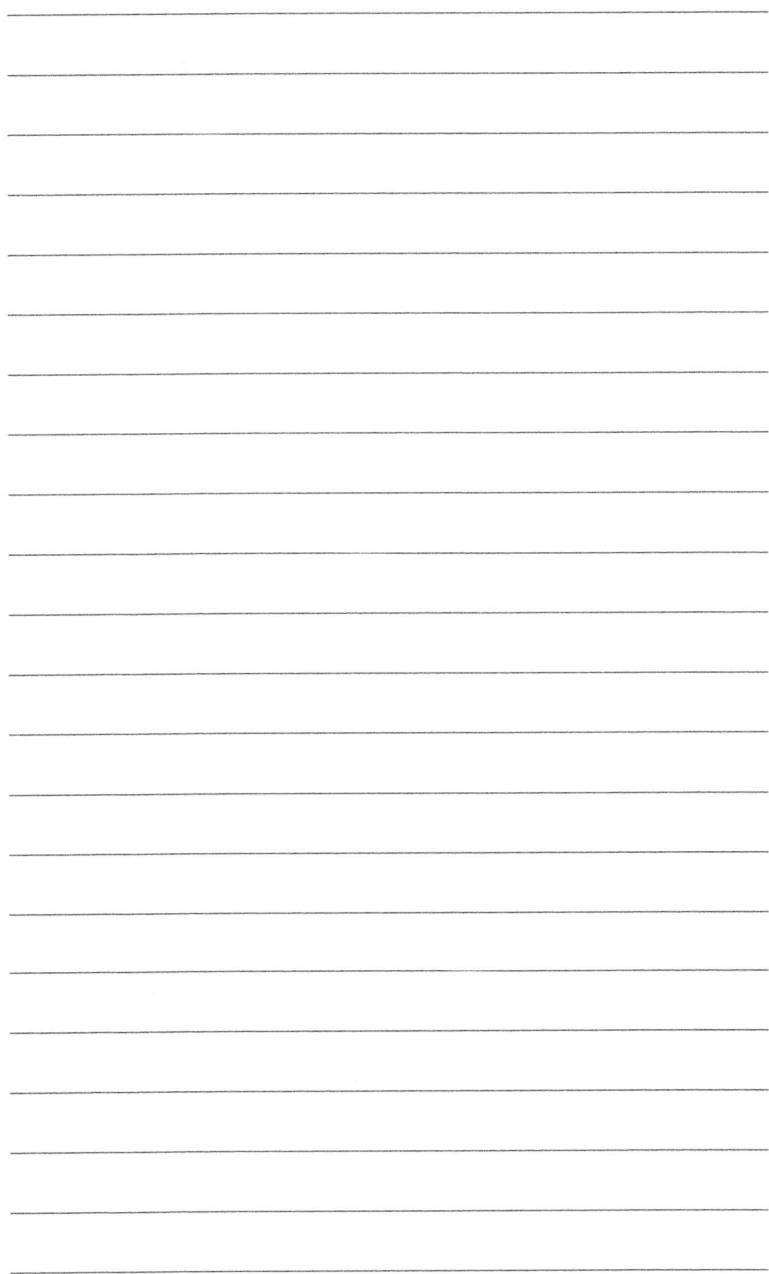

Chapter 3
Urinary Incontinence in Men Post-Prostatectomy

As mentioned in the previous chapters, urinary incontinence is one of the main side effects of prostate cancer surgery, and can profoundly affect men's perception of health, social integration, and overall life satisfaction.

Urinary incontinence can happen with a strong urge to urinate (urge urinary incontinence) or with increased intra-abdominal pressure (stress urinary incontinence).

This chapter will cover changes that may occur after prostate cancer surgery and some theories for why urinary incontinence may occur.

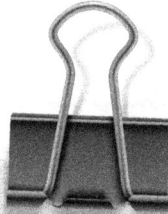

Incontinence and Mental Health

Urinary incontinence and mental health are closely intertwined. Individuals experiencing depression or anxiety are more likely to develop urinary incontinence. Similarly, those with urinary incontinence are prone to experiencing depression or anxiety. This correlation is particularly pertinent for prostate cancer survivors, who are already predisposed to mental health challenges.

Therefore, treating or addressing urinary incontinence after prostate cancer surgery is particularly important and urgent because it may also impact the mental health of these men.

Post-prostatectomy urinary incontinence

The reasons behind post-prostatectomy urinary incontinence are still not widely understood. This chapter aims to elucidate some of the proposed explanations for this phenomenon.

There are many obstacles for urine passage in men **(Fig. 4)**: The sphincters, the prostate itself (as the urethra inside the prostate is narrower) and the long urethra. The bladder has to contract quite forcefully for urination to occur, especially in older males, as the prostate enlarges, narrowing the urethra more.

Fig. 4 Obstacles for urine passage

Before surgery

Prostate

Long urethra

Internal urethral sphincter

External urethral sphincter

After surgery there are fewer obstacles: the urethral tube is shorter, and the prostate gland is removed together with the internal urethral sphincter. The bladder may still be strongly contracting, but now there are fewer obstacles increasing the likelihood of more urinary leakage. Also, if the internal urethral sphincter is removed or damaged, there will be less urethral support and more risk of leakage during activities and/or increased intra-abdominal pressure.

and/or increased intra-abdominal pressure.

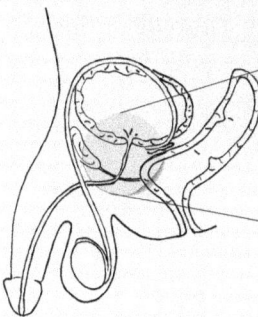

Fig. 4 Obstacles for urine passage

After surgery

Damaged or removed internal urethral sphincter

Shorter urethra

During the first 3 months after surgery there will likely be more leakage and less urinary control while the body is recovering from the surgery. After 3-4 months, urinary incontinence should be improving and spontaneous recovery can be expected after 6-24 months post surgery. A large percentage of males will have minimal or no urinary incontinence after 1 year post surgery.

Stress urinary incontinence (SUI), is spontaneous urine leakage which happens with increased intra-abdominal pressure or movement. Radical Prostatectomy is one of the main causes for SUI in men [6] [7]. Usually, urinary leakage occurs with coughing, sneezing, quick movements, lifting, and certain activities – such as sit-to-stand. Less commonly, men can also leak when a strong urge to urinate occurs. Urge Incontinence will be discussed in the next chapter.

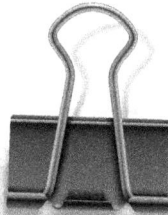

Constant leakage

After radical prostatectomy, a small percentage of men may experience nerve damage or damage directly to the urethral sphincters, leading to decreased closure of the sphincters. Without this closure, urine will be constantly flowing out of the urethra. Natural anatomical closure of the urethral sphincters occurs while seating or lying down enabling urine to be better contained in the bladder. Note however that constant dribbling will likely occur in standing positions.

Although the nerves and urethral sphincters have the capacity to regenerate spontaneously, in some cases, constant leakage can persist permanently. In these situations, it is necessary to seek additional solutions, such as corrective surgeries.

Two common surgical options to treat persistent urinary leakage are artificial sphincters and sling surgery. Artificial sphincters are surgically implanted devices around the urethra to control urine flow, providing artificial closure of the sphincters. On the other hand, sling surgery involves the implantation of a synthetic strip or tape under the urethra to offer support and increase urethral pressure, helping to prevent leaks.

It's important to discuss with your doctor the available surgical options as well as the risks and benefits associated with each procedure to make an informed decision about the most suitable treatment for your condition.

Urinary leakage usually occurs with:

- Coughing
- Sneezing
- Quick movements
- Lifting

and certain activities such as sit-to-stand

Artificial Urethral Sphincter

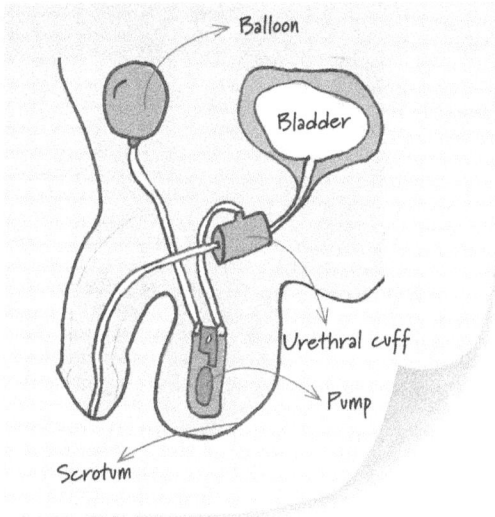

Sling Surgery

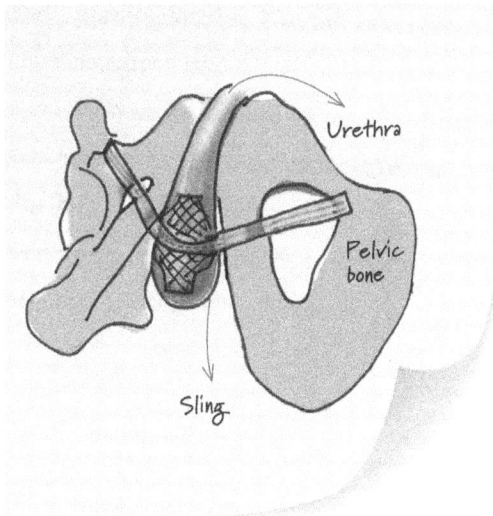

Taking care of your skin

Urine is acidic and can damage your skin, that's why it is important to wash the skin regularly. Pay close attention to any redness, itchiness, or skin sensitivity. If skin is damaged or red, use creams that will cleanse and create a barrier for urine not to penetrate the area before it heals.

Check and see if there is any sensitivity to the incontinent pad or pull-up being worn, as there are many different brands on the market that use non abrasive products. Try to find products that are scent free, and free of alcohol or bleach. Never use toilet paper or tissues as extra layers over the pads as they will not absorb urine properly and will probably contribute to more skin irritation. If you have an open sore that is not healing, consult with your health care practitioner as soon as possible.

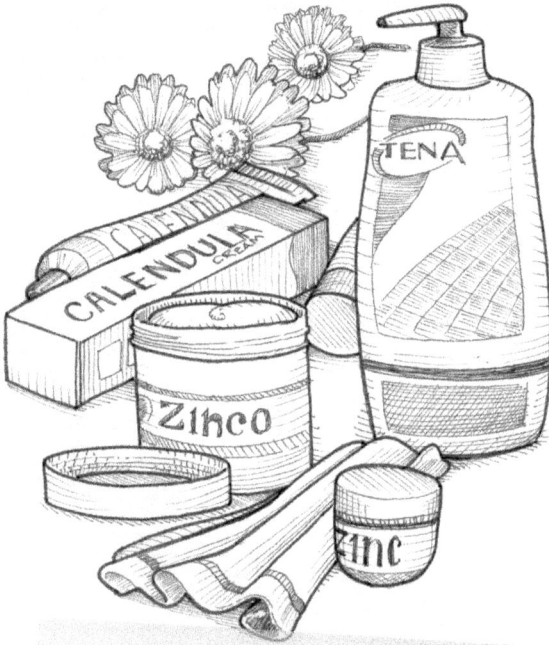

Recommended barrier creams or ointments to protect the skin from irritation caused by urine:

- Zinc oxide formulated to the perineum
- Calendula Cream from Weleda
- Tena cleanse and protect 3 in 1

*Always consult with your physician before using creams.

Notes

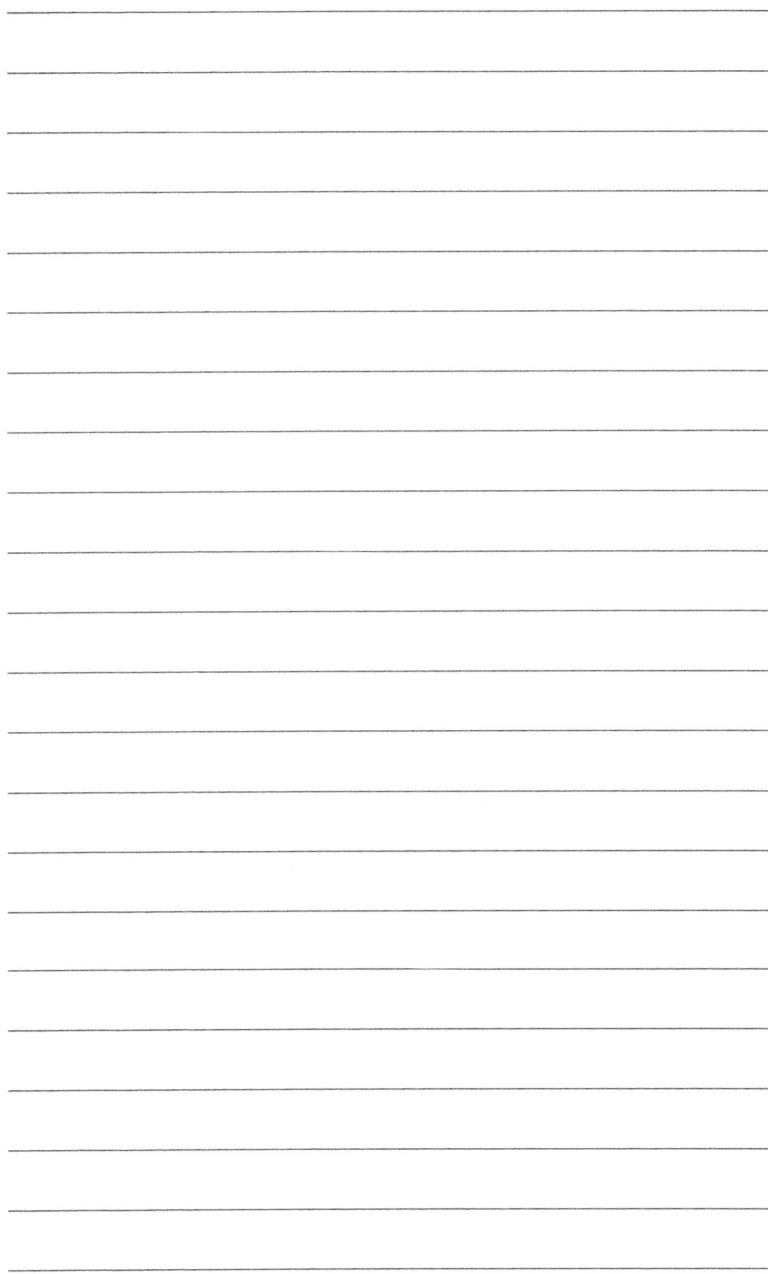

Chapter 4
Urge Urinary Incontinence

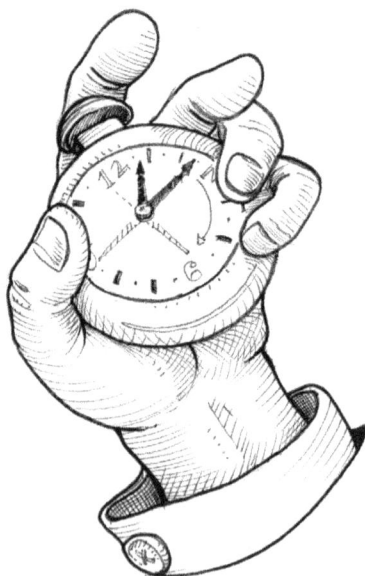

Urge Incontinence accompany with urgency and frequency is commonly seen after prostate cancer surgery.(6) This may result from decreased tension around the sphincter muscles, circulatory and nerve changes, or inflammation resulting from the surgery.(8) Urge incontinence happens with a strong urge to urinate (urgency), and can also be triggered by sensory stimuli, such as running water, putting the keys in the door, or looking at the toilet.

Detrusor instability is when the bladder squeezes randomly causing a strong feeling of urgency to urinate. This can be frustrating because the sudden, strong urgency can make it difficult to hold the urine in, which can be confusing because it occurs even when you know your bladder isn't full. This can cause stress, anxiety, or emotional distress. The best way to control urge incontinence and urgency is to wait until random or strong bladder contractions (strong sensation to urinate) stop before walking or "running" to the washroom. **Remember, the bladder urges come in waves: they start, grow stronger, peak, and then subside.** Calming the bladder before standing up or moving can be the best way to avoid leaking.

Ways to calm the bladder

- If you are walking stop. Sit down if possible.

- Use positive self talk, stay calm and distract yourself from the sensation to urinate.

- Rubbing the back of the thighs or going up on the toes can help relax the bladder **(Appendix 1)**

Another effective technique to help with urgency is by scheduling urination. During the day try to go to the washroom at a set time — for example every 2 hours — until urgency is diminished. Urinary frequency can be monitored by using a Bladder Diary. (Page 142)

Case 1:

A 55-year-old man came to see me with very significant urinary incontinence one year after surgery. He leaked on average 18 times a day. Because he didn't want to wear pads, every time he felt he was going to leak he rushed to the washroom to urinate. Most of his treatment was focused on spacing out urination.

I encouraged him to work on urge suppression techniques and to space urination to at least every 2 hours. After 8 weeks of training, he was only leaking on average 5 times a day and continued to improve thereafter, significantly improving his life satisfaction and urinary control.

Drinking habits can also affect urgency and urge incontinence. If you have urge incontinence, recommendations include:

- Reducing or eliminating caffeine intake
- Drinking water slowly (5 to 8 cups of water a day)
- Reducing or eliminating diuretics such as beer
- Reducing alcohol intake
- Avoiding constipation by eating a high-fiber diet
- Managing stress and anxiety
- **NEVER RUNNING TO THE WASHROOM**

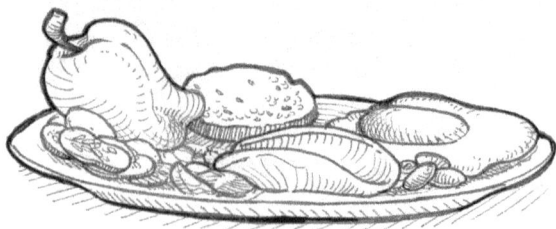

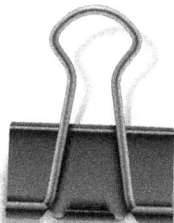

NEVER RUNNING TO
THE WASHROOM

Running to the washroom when you have a strong sensation to urinate is never a good idea! You will be increasing intra-abdominal pressure while the bladder is still contracting and the sphincter muscles are starting to relax. Sit down as soon as you feel a strong urge to urinate. Wait until the sensation diminishes. Then ask yourself:

"Is it time for me to urinate?

"How long has it been since I urinated?"

"Did I ingest a lot of fluid recently?"

"Did I just go to the washroom 30 min ago?"

If it is appropriate to urinate, you still have to have CONTROL. Having control will reduce the chances of urinary incontinence.

Notes

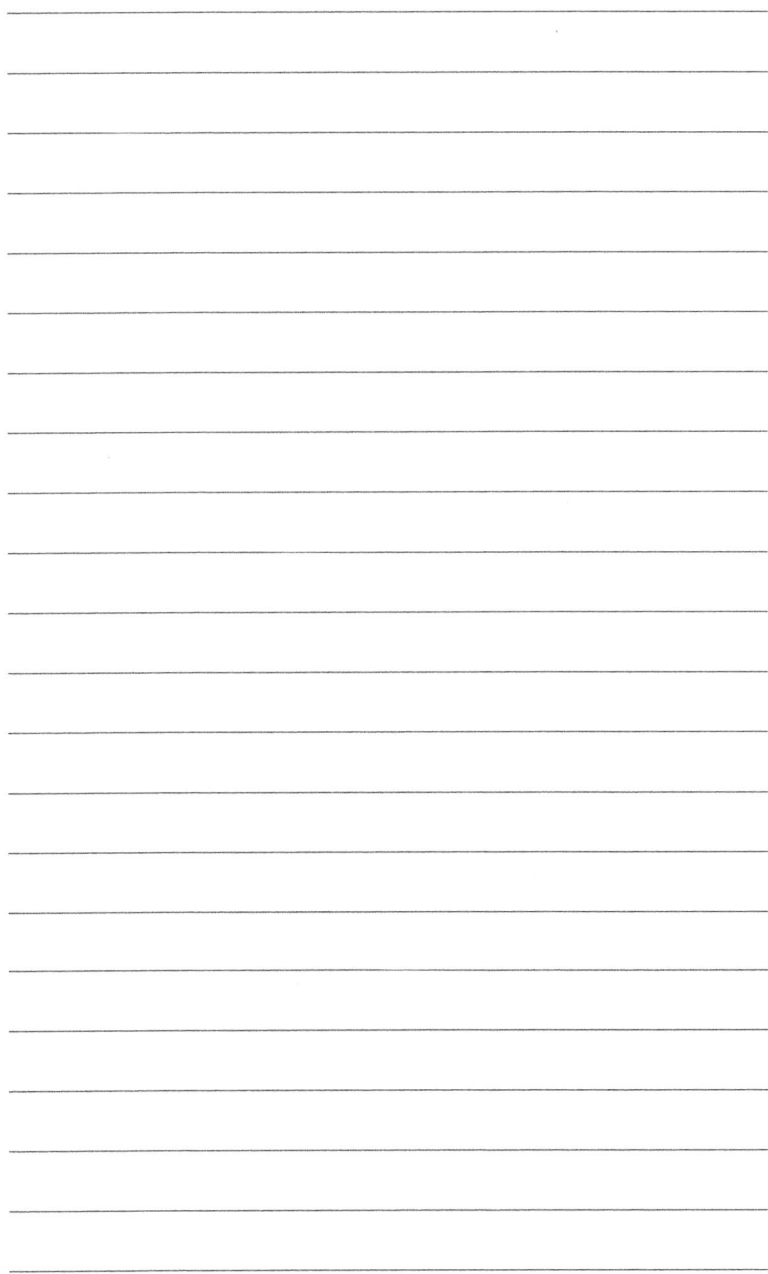

Chapter 5
Bladder Recovery

Urinary incontinence may be present especially during the first 3 months after radical prostatectomy surgery. During the first months after surgery, bladder tissue is repairing itself and consequentially bladder function may be impaired. The bladder is familiarizing itself to its new environment, learning not to contract as forcefully for urination to occur as there are fewer obstacles for urine passage after the surgery. Also, the bladder may still be swollen after surgery, which can affect its fluid capacity.

The severity of urinary leakages will be dependent on many factors; for example, the size of the cancer and tissue involvement, the individual's overall health status prior to surgery, and the surgeon's experience.

Urinary Incontinence can greatly affect men's quality of life (9). Clinically is not uncommon to see men frustrated and unhappy with their slow bladder recovery, and therefore start adopting detrimental behaviours.

Being concerned about leaking-men may:

1. Increase urination frequency

2. Decrease water intake

3. Wake up many times at night to urinate

1. Increasing urination frequency

To try and prevent leakage, men may urinate more frequently. This will not allow the bladder to accumulate normal volume. By not allowing the bladder to stretch, the automatic relationship between the bladder muscles and the sphincters is weakened. By weakening this relationship, there may be more likelihood of urinary incontinence. During the healing phase it is important to maintain and strengthen the bladder/sphincter relationship so the process of urination and urine control can occur naturally.

Try to drink fluids slowly and allow at least 2 hours in-between urinations. Once urinary incontinence improves, men should try to wait 3 to 4 hours in-between urinations.

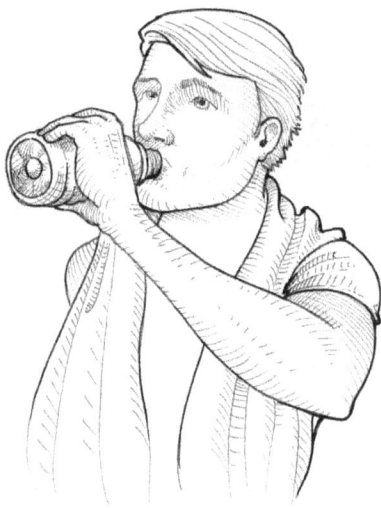

2. Decreasing water intake

Concerned about leaking, men may stop drinking (especially water). This results in the urine being too concentrated and will therefore irritate the bladder lining. This irritation will cause the bladder to contract more often, which triggers the sensation to urinate more often, lowering urine volume and flow. When the bladder is not stretched enough, its contraction is not as strong, resulting in difficulty emptying the bladder. It is therefore important to keep drinking water slowly, to keep urine diluted, and encouraging normal urine volume and flow.

3. Night urination

During sleep, men will have better urine control. Actually, men will start to experience dryness during the night when sleeping. During the first few months after the surgery, men will be afraid to leak during the night and may wake up multiple times to urinate. The sensation to urinate will happen more at night as it will be easier to store urine and for the bladder to stretch. During sleep, the forces of gravity are decreased and lessen the chances of urinary incontinence. Also, there is very little movement during sleep, decreasing the chances of experiencing SUI. Sleep is very important for the process of recovery, so it is recommended to train the bladder to be less active at night. Increasing sleep time will also help to re-train bladder capacity and urine control. The optimal goal is to wake up only once, or to try to sleep through the night without urinating.

To help control strong urges to urinate during the night, stop drinking fluids 2 to 3 hours before bed time and avoid caffeine or diuretics in the evenings.

Drinking most of your fluids during the day will make you less thirsty at night.

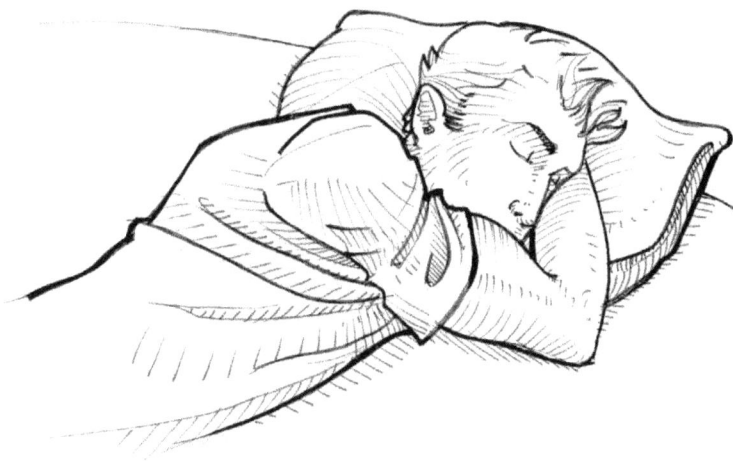

Notes

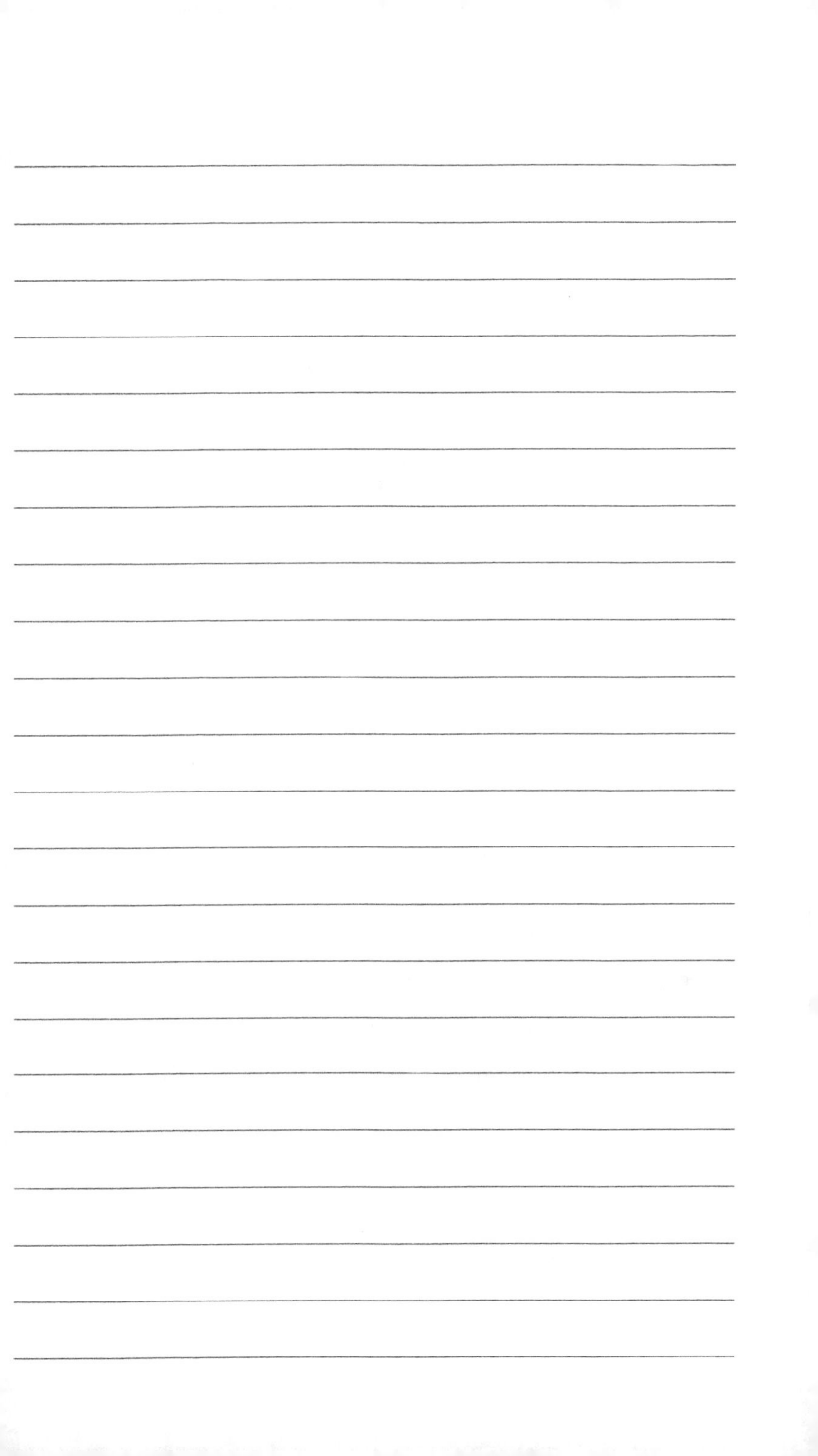

Chapter 6
The Milking Technique

After surgery, the bladder will sit lower than before putting more pressure on the urethra. The urethra is the hollow tube that carries urine from the bladder to the outer orifice. After urinating, a few drops may remain inside the tube due to the anatomical shift that may happen after the surgery **(Fig. 5)**. Usually when this happens leakage occurs right after urination when moving or changing position, such as when pulling up the underwear and/ or pants. This type of incontinence is called post-voidal dribble.

There are 3 methods of removing urine that remains in the urethra:

1. Moving the hand from the base of the penis out towards the orifice (clearing the tube)

2. Elevating the scrotum to help ease urine passage

3. Squeezing the pelvic floor muscles after urinating

Fig. 5

Post-voidal Residual

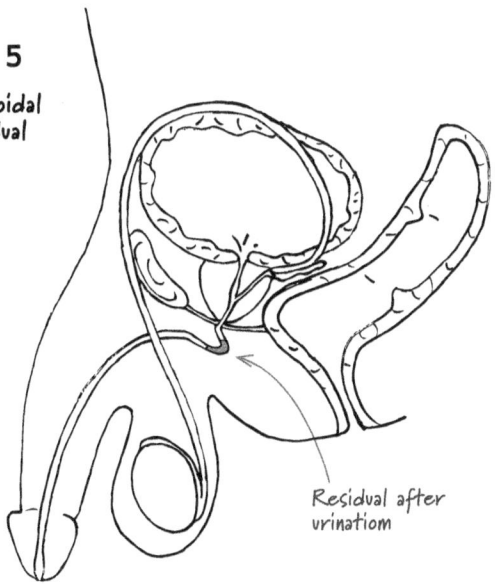

Residual after urinatiom

Notes

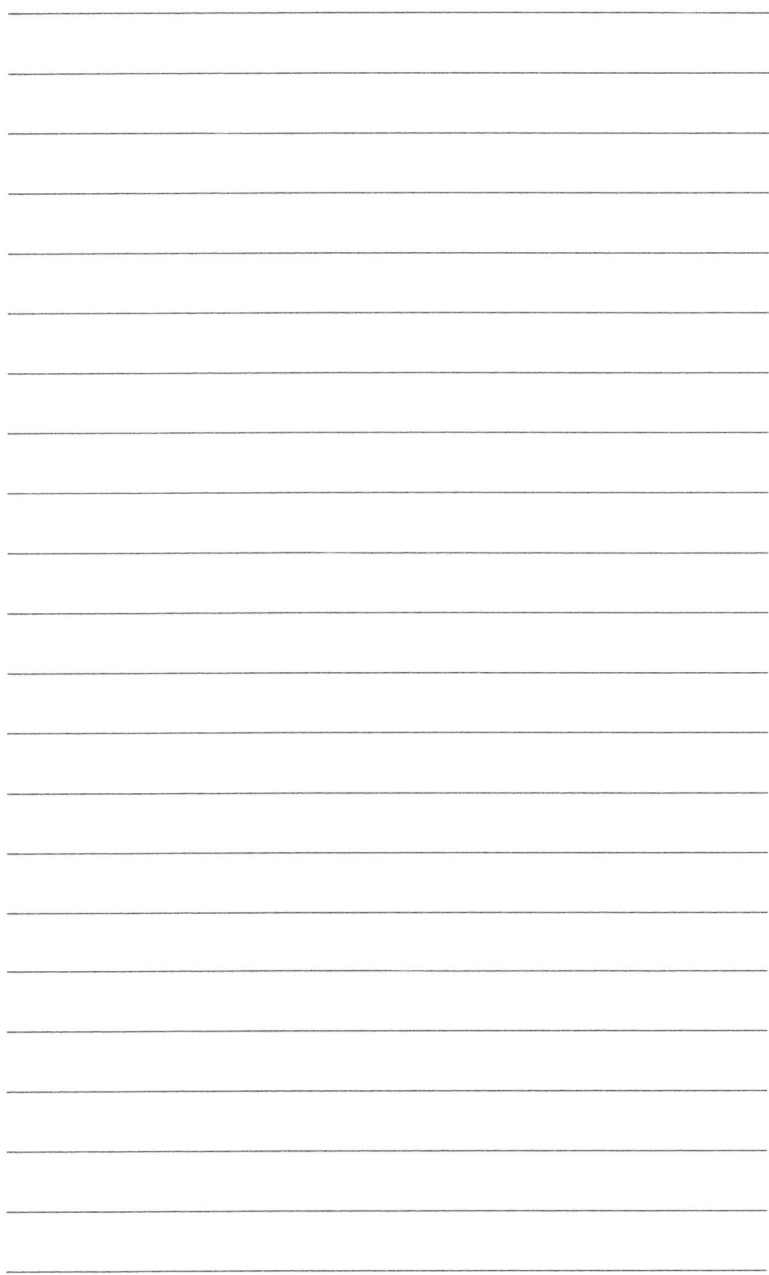

Chapter 7
Bowels and Diet

Constipation can be one of the main contributors to urinary incontinence. The bowels (large intestine) sit very close to the bladder, and if there is stool impaction, it will press on the bladder, increasing intra-abdominal pressure and incontinence. Constipation can also cause urgency and frequency, due to constant bladder pressure.

Avoiding constipation by maintaining a high-fibre diet and drinking 6-8 glasses of water a day can help reduce incontinence. The stools should be formed but soft and easily passed. For more information on managing constipation please refer to **Appendix 2**.

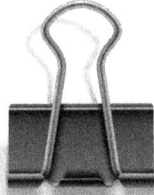

Useful tip post surgery

Even if constipation is not an issue for you, after surgery you may experience difficulties passing stool due to pain medication side effects. Make sure not to strain to pass stool especially right after surgery as it can potentially interfere with recovery. Stool softeners and mild laxatives can help you keep stool consistency during the first few days after surgery. Make sure to consult with your physician first before taking any constipation medication.

Notes

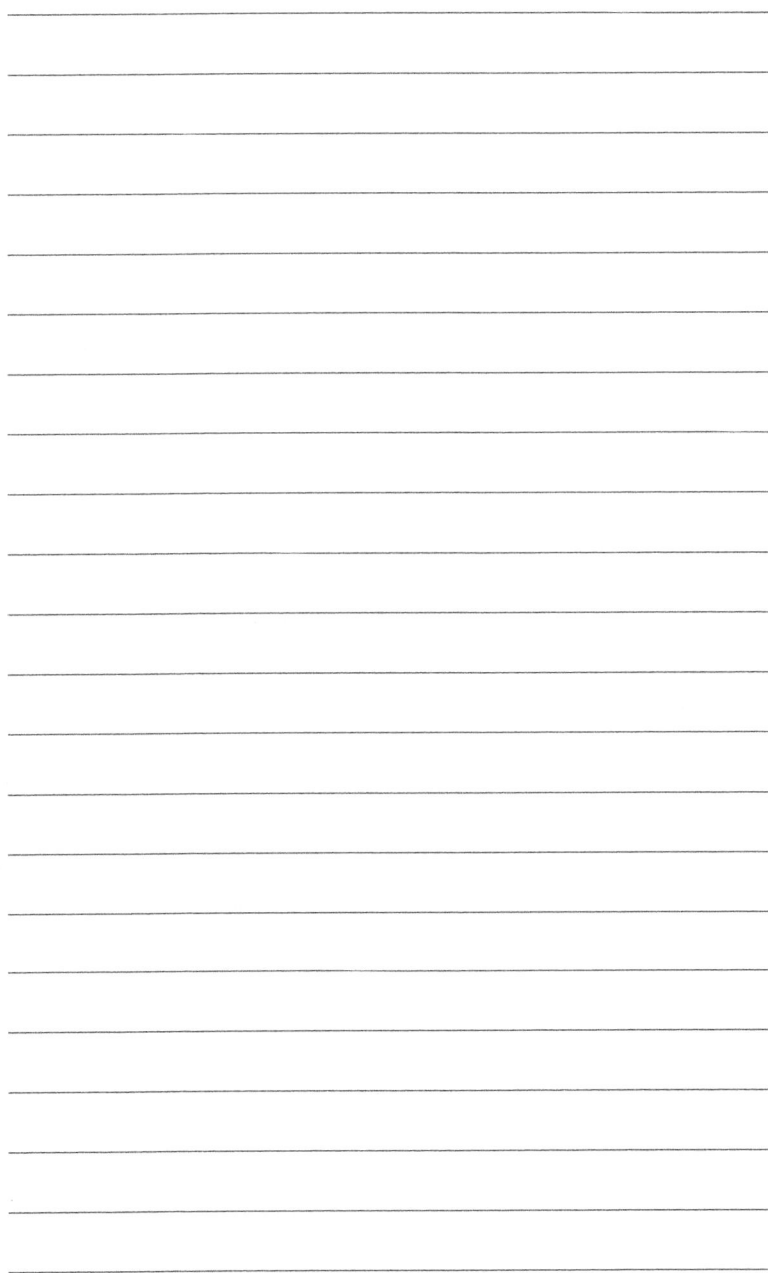

Chapter 8

Pelvic Floor Muscle Training

The pelvic floor muscles are postural muscles located on the lower pelvis supporting the bladder and the rectum in males. They attach from the tailbone to the pubic bone and act as a sling to support the pelvis **(Fig. 6)**. They are "small muscles" as they can increase or decrease in activity depending on the individual activity level. For example: If someone is lying down and not moving, the pelvic floor muscles have minimal activity, however, if someone is running or hiking the pelvic floor muscles will be more active.

The pelvic floor muscles also have an important role in preventing urinary leakages. When the pelvic floor muscles contract they clamp the urethra closed preventing urine loss during coughing, sneezing, or any time intra-abdominal pressure increases.

If pelvic floor muscles are weak, too tight, or lack coordination, they won't contract at the right time, resulting in potential urinary incontinence. Pelvic floor muscle training is essential to help improve urinary incontinence in men post-prostatectomy.

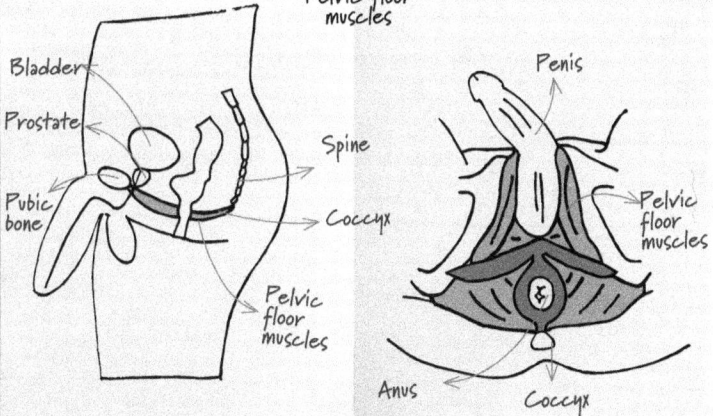

Fig. 6
Pelvic floor muscles

Bladder
Prostate
Pubic bone
Spine
Coccyx
Pelvic floor muscles
Penis
Pelvic floor muscles
Anus
Coccyx

There is increasing evidence that pelvic floor muscle training can help treat urinary incontinence (UI) in men post radical prostatectomy surgery, especially if the training starts before surgery (10, 11). Please note that pelvic floor muscle training is not just about strengthening the pelvic floor muscles! This cannot be emphasized enough! Men have to be able to first learn how to correctly activate the muscles and to acquire proper muscle coordination; such as learning how to effectively contract and relax the pelvic floor muscles before starting a strengthening program.

The pelvic floor muscles need to have fast reflex reactions to prevent leakages once abdominal pressure increases, such as with coughing, sneezing, and lifting heavy weights. In summary, if pelvic floor muscles are strong, but have poor coordination and poor relaxation, urinary control will not be achieved.

Here are the steps to be followed for optimal pelvic floor muscle recovery:

- step 1 – Pelvic Floor Muscle Activation (recruitment)

- step 2 – Pelvic Floor Muscle Coordination and Relaxation

- step 3 – Pelvic Floor Muscle Strengthening

- step 4 – Functional Pelvic Floor Muscle Training

Step 1. Pelvic Floor Muscle Activation (recruitment)

Pelvic floor muscle activation (or recruitment) refers to isolating the contractions of the pelvic floor muscles. The first thing to learn is how to contract the pelvic muscles independently, without using other muscles in the body.

Try this exercise in a comfortable lying position with the knees bent. Think about the area between the anus and scrotum. How does that area feel? Is there tension around the anus? If so, can this tension be relieved?

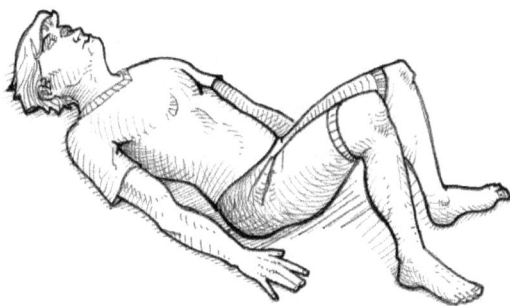

When the anus and the perineal area is relaxed, there is a feeling as if the anus is more open and gas could be liberated without resistance. Stay in this relaxed position for a few minutes then try to contract your pelvic muscles by visualizing the muscles and area between the anus and the scrotum. The pelvic floor muscles are a sling of muscles attached from the pubic bone to the tail bone, so when they are contracted the pelvic organs move upward. In men post-prostatectomy, new evidence suggests that it is very important to activate the muscles around the urethra and the anterior part of the pelvic floor muscles. Therefore, a useful cue to employ is "shortening the penis" or stopping urine flow. The stronger the contraction, the more movement will be sensed inside the pelvis and at the base of the penis. However, the movement sensation is small compared to other parts of the body.

When isolating the contraction of the pelvic floor muscles, the rest of body should not move, so try not to contract the higher abdominal muscles, gluteus muscles, or leg muscles. Breathe normally, and do not hold your breath. Hold this contraction for a few seconds then relax.

Step 2. Pelvic Floor Muscle Coordination and Relaxation

Coordination of the pelvic floor muscles is achieved when the muscles can be effectively contracted and relaxed. Relaxation makes up of over 50% of pelvic floor muscle training - muscles cannot contract if they are not first relaxed.

Think about the quality of the contraction of the pelvic floor muscles. Is the contraction smooth and are the contractions being sustained for a few seconds before they are released? When relaxation occurs, can the sensation of downward movement be experienced successfully? How long does it take for complete relaxation to be experienced? If it takes a long time for relaxation to occur, it is suggested to wait longer before attempting another contraction. Rest for at least 3 times longer than the contraction hold.

For example

For a 3-second hold, the rest phase would be 9–10 seconds. But if relaxation occurs only after 30 seconds then wait 30–60 seconds before contracting the pelvic muscles again.

Teaching muscles to relax can be challenging, so it is very important that relaxation can be achieved before continuing to Step 3.

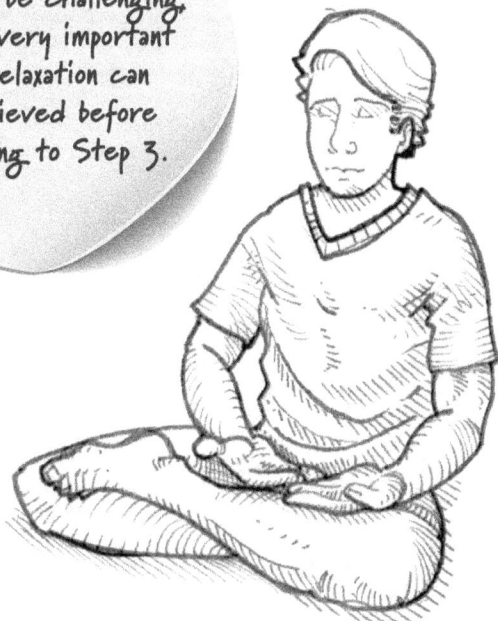

Step 3. Pelvic Floor Muscle Strengthening

Now that muscle activation and coordination have been achieved, the next step will be to improve pelvic floor muscle strength. The goal of the strengthening program is to increase muscle bulk (hypertrophy) and to elevate the bladder neck, making it easier to control leakages. But remember not everyone needs a strengthening program, as some men can manage their symptoms by following a relaxation program.

Muscles have to constantly be challenged in order to keep increasing in size and strength. The goal is to try to achieve maximum pelvic floor muscle contraction.

Try to hold maximum contraction for about 3-5 seconds and fully relax between contractions for at least 3 times the holding time. Try 7-10 repetitions, but make sure to stop before you notice muscle fatigue. (Note that when muscles start to fatigue the contractions become weaker). Most importantly, all of the contractions should have the same strength. Stop exercising when noticing the contractions are becoming weaker, or that other muscles are starting to contract instead. Don't exercise more than 3 times a day, as the muscles need to rest and recover.

To continue to challenge pelvic floor muscles, change positions and use gravity as resistance. The optimal goal is to achieve PASSIVE SUPPORT from the muscles, meaning the muscles are thick and strong enough to increase pelvic organ support and function.

Just remember that each individual requires a personalized program. Therefore, it is imperative to consult with a pelvic health physical therapist before commencing any home program for a proper examination and to facilitate progress in exercises.

THESE EXERCISES ARE NOT EASY TO DO. YOU MUST CONCENTRATE AND ALLOCATE TIME TO DO THEM PROPERLY.

EXAMPLE OF PROGRESSIONS

LYING WITH KNEES BENT
(gravity assisting the pelvic floor muscle contraction)

LYING LEGS FLAT OR APART
(gravity being eliminated)

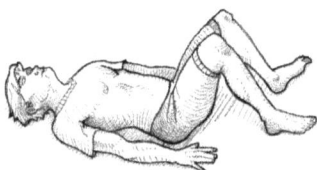

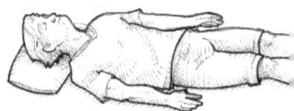

Easier

Beginning with easiest

SITTING
(gravity adding weight to challenge pelvic floor muscle contraction)

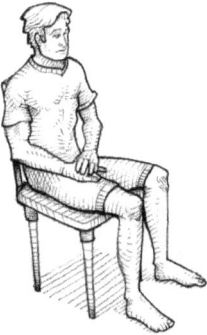

STANDING
(gravity plus body weight increasing the challenge of pelvic floor muscle contraction)

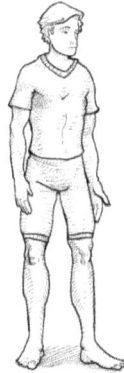

Harder

Step 4. Functional Program

Once muscles are coordinated and strong, there are circumstances in which pelvic floor muscles could be used functionally. For example, if needed, pelvic floor muscles can be contracted gently just before coughing, sneezing or heavy lifting, to prevent urinary leakages.

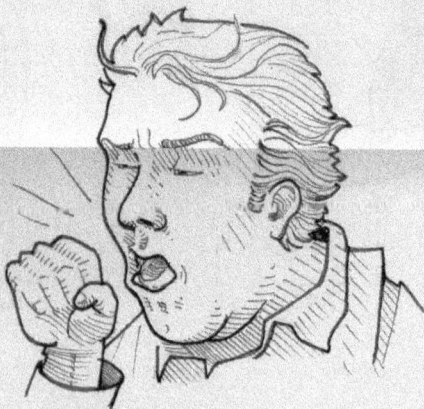

Remember, the pelvic floor muscle contractions should be short and with optimal relaxation. The idea is to train pelvic floor muscle reflex reaction, encouraging an increase in tension on the urethral sphincter (the valve which controls incontinence) before increased intra-abdominal pressure.

It is recommended to have the pelvic floor muscles checked by a pelvic health physical therapist before starting a home program. These are not easy exercises. The sensation experienced by pelvic floor muscle contraction can be very small, and if someone has difficulties with relaxation these exercises are not recommended until relaxation, is learned and achieved. Note that only a small percentage of men can perform these exercises correctly at first.

Pre-prostatectomy pelvic floor training

Dr. Jo Milios introduced a novel approach to train the pelvic floor muscles pre-prostatectomy, which demonstrated improvements in post-prostatectomy urinary incontinence. (11)

Her program involved training the "fast twitch fibers" by rapidly contracting and relaxing the anterior part of the pelvic floor muscles (utilizing cues such as "shortening the penis") for 10 repetitions, and training the slow twitch fibers by **gently** contracting around the urethra for 10 seconds and relaxing for 10 seconds times 10. These two types of exercises were repeated 6 times a day, with progression to a standing position.

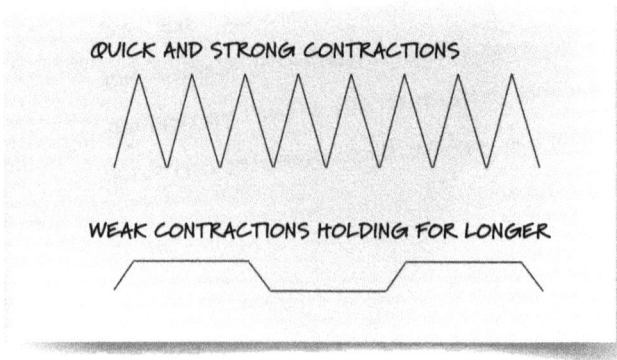

QUICK AND STRONG CONTRACTIONS

WEAK CONTRACTIONS HOLDING FOR LONGER

The objective of a pre-prostatectomy program is to enhance the condition of the muscles prior to surgery, aiming for a faster return to continence. Pre-rehabilitation, under the supervision of a physical therapist, serves the additional purpose of assessing and screening for other symptoms, such as urgency and mental health status, which could potentially delay the recovery process.

Strategies to facilitate contraction of the anterior pelvic floor muscles

- Use cues such as "shortening the penis" or "pinching in the urethra."

- Lean forward while sitting on a chair

- Shift the weight of the body forward onto the feet when practicing in a standing posture.

Notes

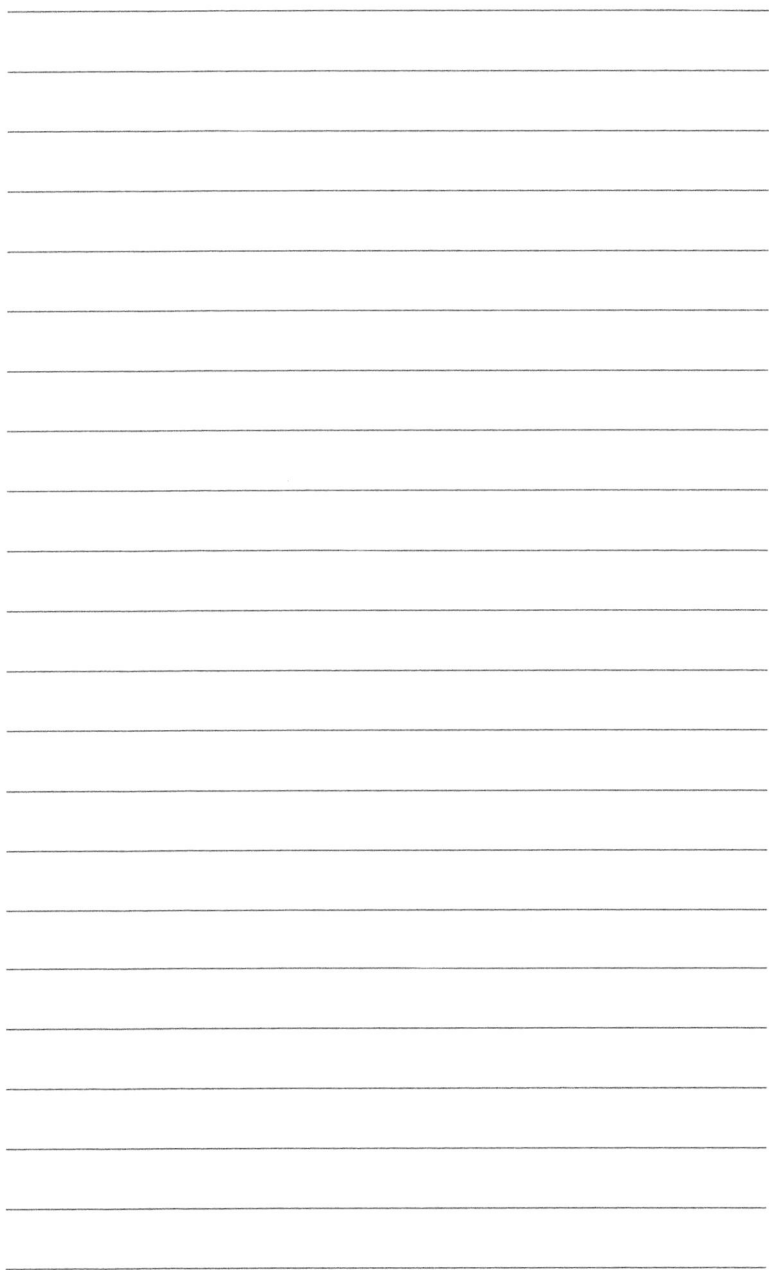

Chapter 9
Relaxation

Relaxation is such an important topic that it has a chapter of its own. It is very important to learn pelvic floor muscle relaxation before any type of pelvic floor muscle training or "Kegel" exercises. Pelvic Floor Muscle Training is not recommended if there is difficulty relaxing the pelvic floor muscles, because it can be associated with bladder dysfunction (12).

Clinically, relaxation is a very prominent issue. Most of the time, men are not even aware that they have pelvic floor muscle relaxation difficulties, and most of the time it can only be discovered during a pelvic floor muscle evaluation.

Clients with non-relaxing pelvic floor muscles may show signs of:

- Pelvic pain or pelvic discomfort
- Urgency and frequency
- Urinary incontinence which happens mostly in the afternoon or evening
- Urinary incontinence which happens randomly, especially after strenuous activities (but not during the activities)
- Difficulties urinating or defecating

Treatment for non-relaxing pelvic floor muscles may include:

- Mind-Body Quieting
- Diaphragmatic breathing (Appendix 3)
- Lower body stretches and "opening" postures (Appendix 4)
- Pelvic Floor muscle Biofeedback treatment usually performed in the clinic, or at home with a biofeedback hand held machine (Chapter 11 - Case2)

Mind-Body Quieting

Excessive pelvic floor muscle resting tone and increased activity level of bladder and bowel contractions can be decreased through physiological quieting of the body and mind.

Find a quiet warm room with a chair or bed that gives complete support from your head to your feet. Use pillows to support your neck, lower back, arms and knees, or wherever is needed for comfort. Then:

1. Focus on your breathing and feel your breathing pattern, then let your abdomen rise when inhaling and fall when exhaling.

2. Feeling the support of the bed or chair, relax from the top of your head to the tips of your toes.

3. Focusing on your face and neck, notice where there is tension or tightness, and where there is quiet and calmness. Then say to yourself 3 to 4 times – "my face and neck muscles are quiet and calm, my face and neck muscles are calmer and calmer."

4. Proceed from head to toe in the same manner, focusing on each body part as you did the face and neck. Relax the right and left arms and hand muscles. Keep relaxing down your spine. Relax your chest and abdomen. Relax your gluteus muscles. Relax right and left legs and feet all the way down to your toes.

5. After the entire body is relaxed, go back to your pelvic area and relax your pelvic and anal muscles.

6. Maintain mind-body quietness for 10-20 min.

One or two 20-minute mind-body quieting sessions a day are recommended, ideally early afternoon to help with urinary incontinence that happens in the later afternoon or evenings.

Usually diaphragmatic breathing can be practiced 3 times a day for about 10-15 minutes each time.

These are very safe exercises to do even before seeing a trained physiotherapist for pelvic floor muscle evaluation.

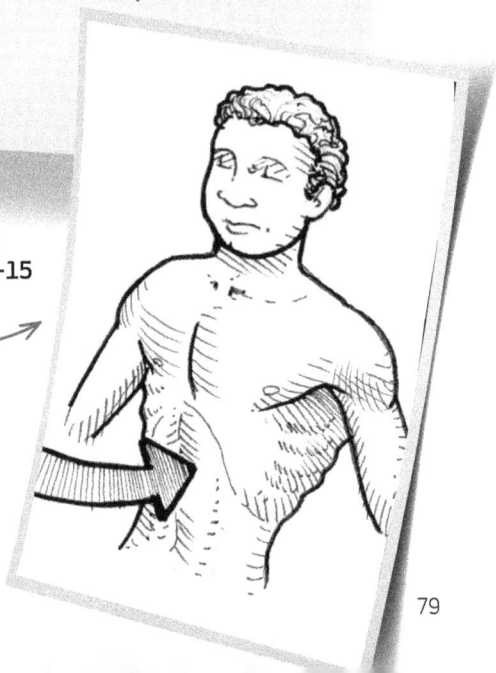

Notes

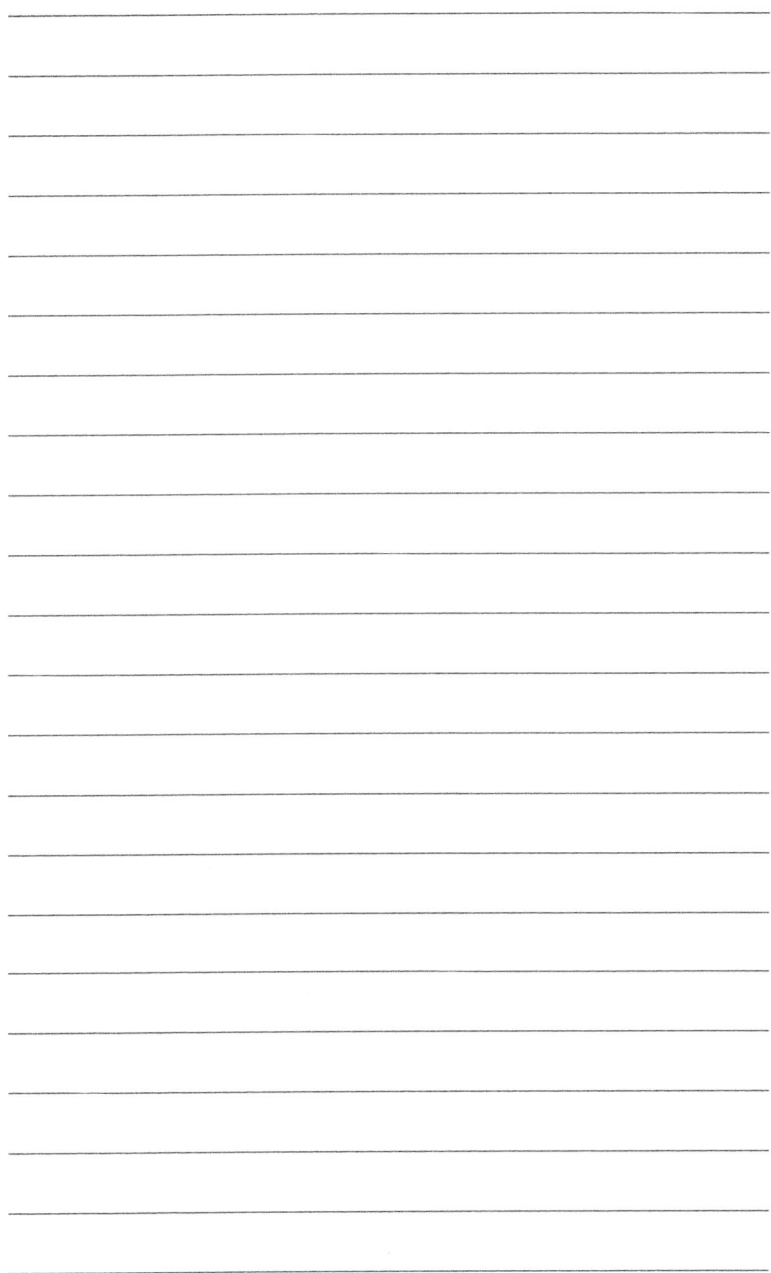

Chapter 10
Emotional Health

An emotion is a state of feeling, or a conscious mental reaction that happens throughout the day. It is transitional - it should come and go. It is normal to feel sad, angry and frustrated, especially after a life threatening condition and surgery with life-changing side effects. If emotions are affecting physical well-being, such as changes in mood, sleep, intimacy and relationships, then emotional health should be addressed.

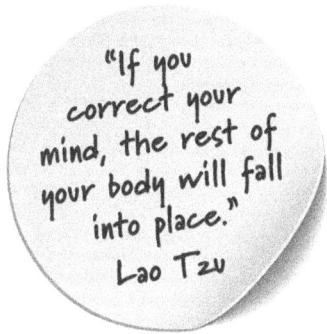

It is important to address emotional health the same way physical health is addressed. As explained in the previous chapter, bladder function is controlled by the nervous system, and if the nervous system is affected by emotional distress, then normal bladder function will be impaired.

There is a strong relationship between mental health status and urinary impairment. In the older adult population, depression and urinary incontinence can be closely related to each other (13). Prostate cancer survivors are particularly vulnerable to developing mental disorders such as depression or anxiety due to the life-altering effects of cancer diagnosis and treatment, challenges which can significantly impact their recovery and overall quality of life.

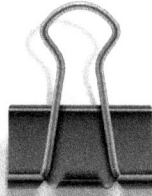

Stress

Stress can also interfere with physical health. Stress can depress mental activity in the higher centers of the brain. During stress, the more primitive brain area is stimulated (hypothalamus), which makes people operate in survival mode. Over time this can be detrimental as it interferes with sleep, short-term memory, logical thinking, cardiac function, and overall sense of well being. Relaxation, deep breathing techniques, physical activity, and social support can counter the stress response and accelerate the process of normalizing body function (14).

The bladder as an emotional organ

The bladder can function as an 'emotional' organ, reacting to stress and anxiety; for instance, symptoms like urinary urgency frequency and pain can worsen.

For example, when someone is worried about something or anxious about being late, they may feel the need to urinate even though the bladder is not actually full. Consequently, the bladder will contract in response to these emotions. If emotions remain unchanged or if stress becomes chronic, it is possible that the bladder will become more reactive over time, and symptoms of incontinence become worse.

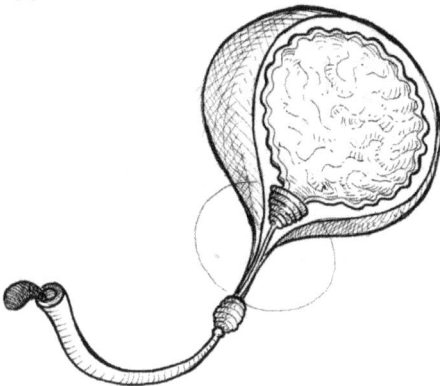

The pelvic stress reflex

The pelvic floor muscles can be highly reactive. It Has been demostrated that these muscles contract in response to stress.

In clinical practice and research, it's widely recognized that many pelvic issues can be triggered by stressful events. When muscles become reactive, their quality and response can change over time, leading to symptoms such as urinary, sexual problems and pain.

Practices that may improve mental wellness

- Mindfulness
- Yoga Practices
- Medical Qigong
- Regular Physical Activities
- Psychosocial therapy / counselling

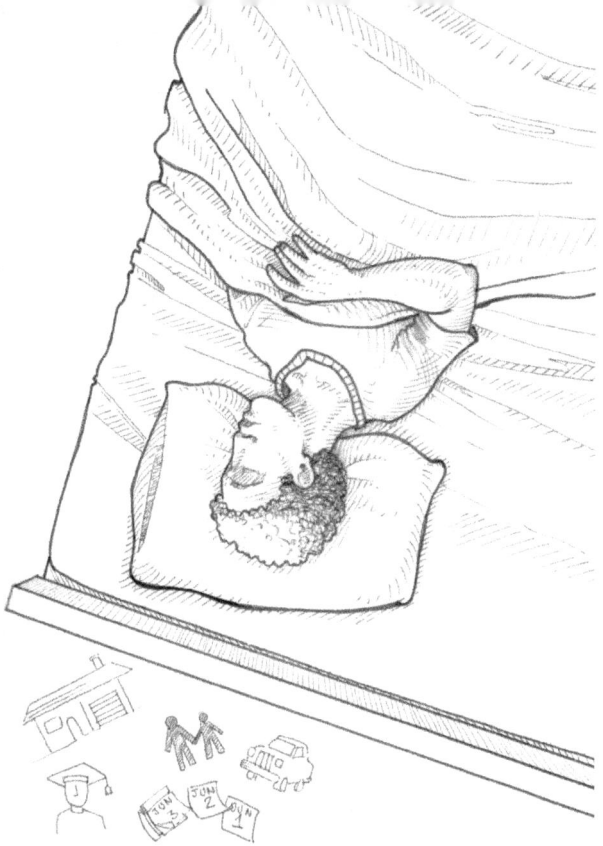

Ultimately, the crucial initial step is to recognize any changes and dysfunction in emotional or mental health, and then take proactive steps towards treatment options. It's important to discuss these changes with your healthcare provider or seek assistance from a mental health clinician. Addressing emotional and mental health issues can significantly aid in bladder and sexual recovery.

Notes

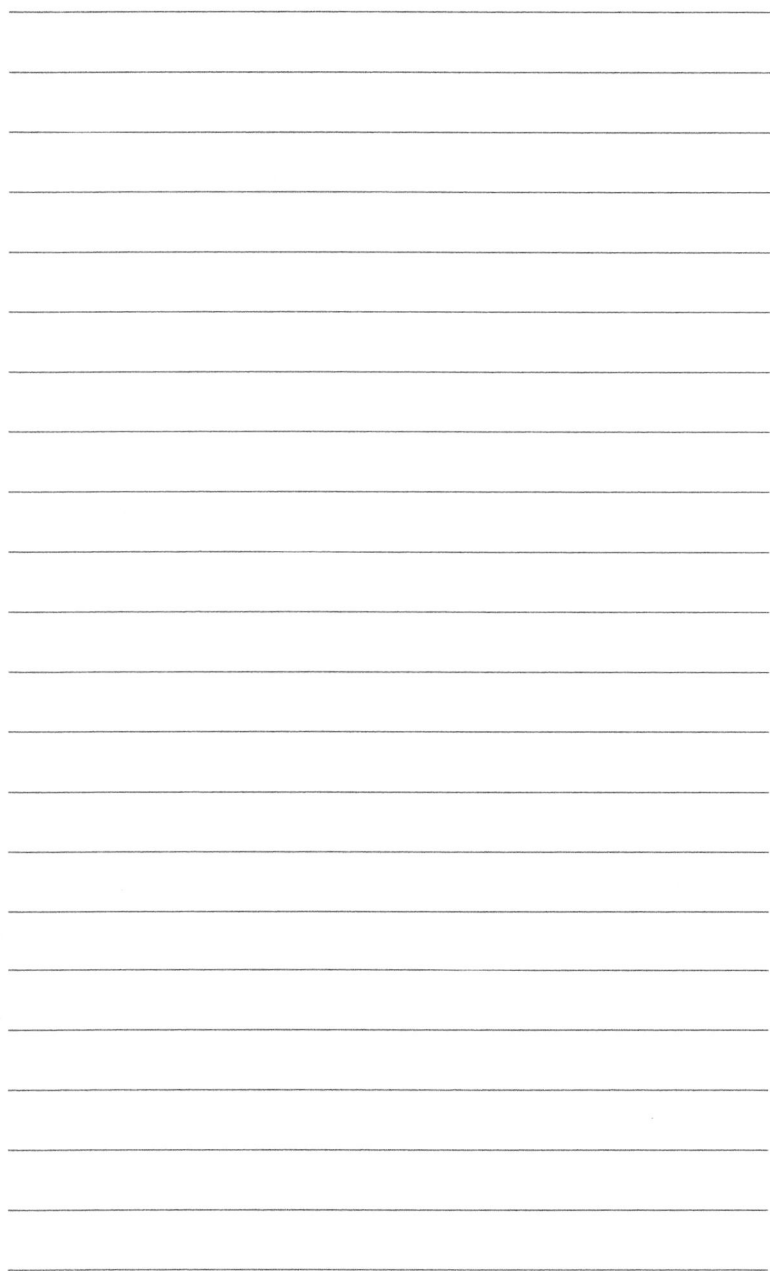

Chapter 11
Erectile Function

Recent studies suggest that being proactive about the penis, such as penile rehabilitation, may help increase the chances of future erections post-prostatectomy (15). Most of the time, erectile dysfunction occurs once the cavernous nerve is compressed or cut, resulting in lack of blood flow to the penis. Even if the nerve is spared during the surgery, the swelling around the nerve can cause temporary nerve damage that can take up to 4 years to regenerate (16). The idea of penile rehabilitation early after surgery is to maintain and preserve penile length and tissue, so once the nerve is regenerated, the penile tissue is healthy and can continue to expand during increased blood flow. Penile massage (expanding and contracting the penis for 10-15 times) and the use of a penile pump 3-4 times a week is recommended as a form to maintain penile length and girth during recovery time. For those who have undergone nerve-sparing procedures, it is crucial to initiate penile rehabilitation as soon as possible, before permanent changes occur to the tissue. Some medications such as Cialis or Viagra, that increase blood flow to the penis, can also be prescribed by your physician, but it is still debatable if these medications will improve erectile dysfunction post-prostatectomy [17].

Other than penile pumps and medications, intracavernosal injections can also be utilized as an effective method to promote sufficient erections for penetration, and they can be administered as early as 8-9 weeks post-op for certain individuals. [18]

Remember that men will always be sexual beings, even if suffering from erectile dysfunction! Intimacy and orgasm can still be obtained without erections. Consulting with sex therapists, urologists or sexual health educators is recommended to address sexual dysfunctions. Psychological factors for sexual dysfunction should be considered and the men's partners should be involved whenever possible [19].

Pelvic Floor Muscle Training can also help improve sexual function in males [20].

Remember that men will always be sexual beings, even if suffering from erectile dysfunction!

Case 2:

I had been seeing a client with a history of erectile dysfunction that came to see me to learn pelvic floor muscles exercises before his prostatectomy surgery. I noticed during his assessment that he had difficulties relaxing his pelvic floor muscle, so I recommended biofeedback treatment. His pelvic floor muscle tone was very high at rest, so most of his treatment was about relaxation and pelvic floor muscle relaxation awareness. His resting pelvic floor muscle tone decreased, and he noticed improvement in his erections since he started the relaxation exercises.

This case shows that pelvic floor muscle relaxation dysfunction can also play a role in men's sexual function.

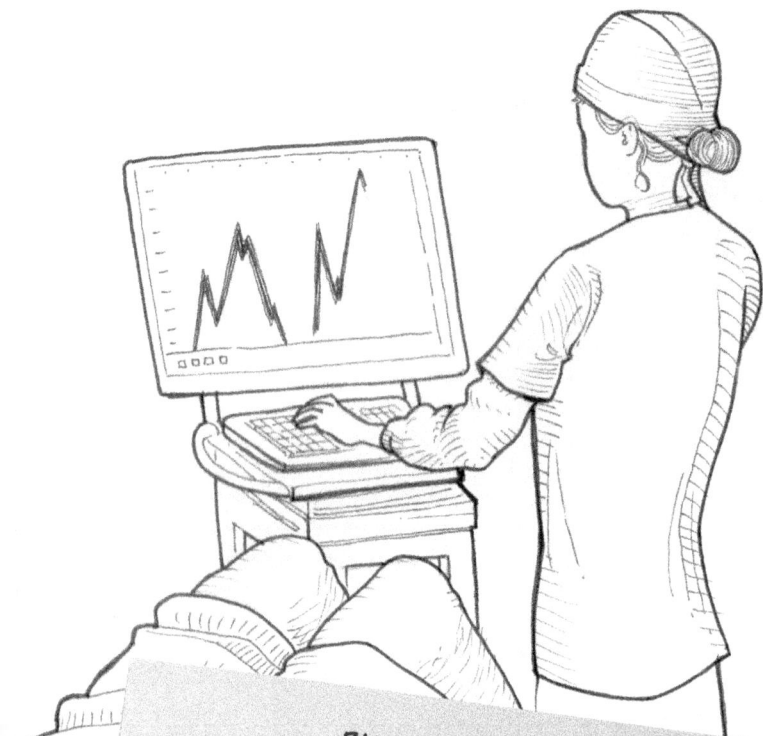

BIOFEEDBACK

Biofeedback is an effective way to learn to relax the pelvic floor muscles. The pelvic floor muscle activity is seen on a computer screen to facilitate learning and improve pelvic floor muscle awareness. It is a painless procedure that uses special sensors connected to the pelvic floor muscles (internally or externally) and a computer monitor. Over time, this "feedback" mechanism helps to connect with the pelvic floor muscles and learn the sensation of pelvic floor muscle relaxation, especially at rest.

Notes

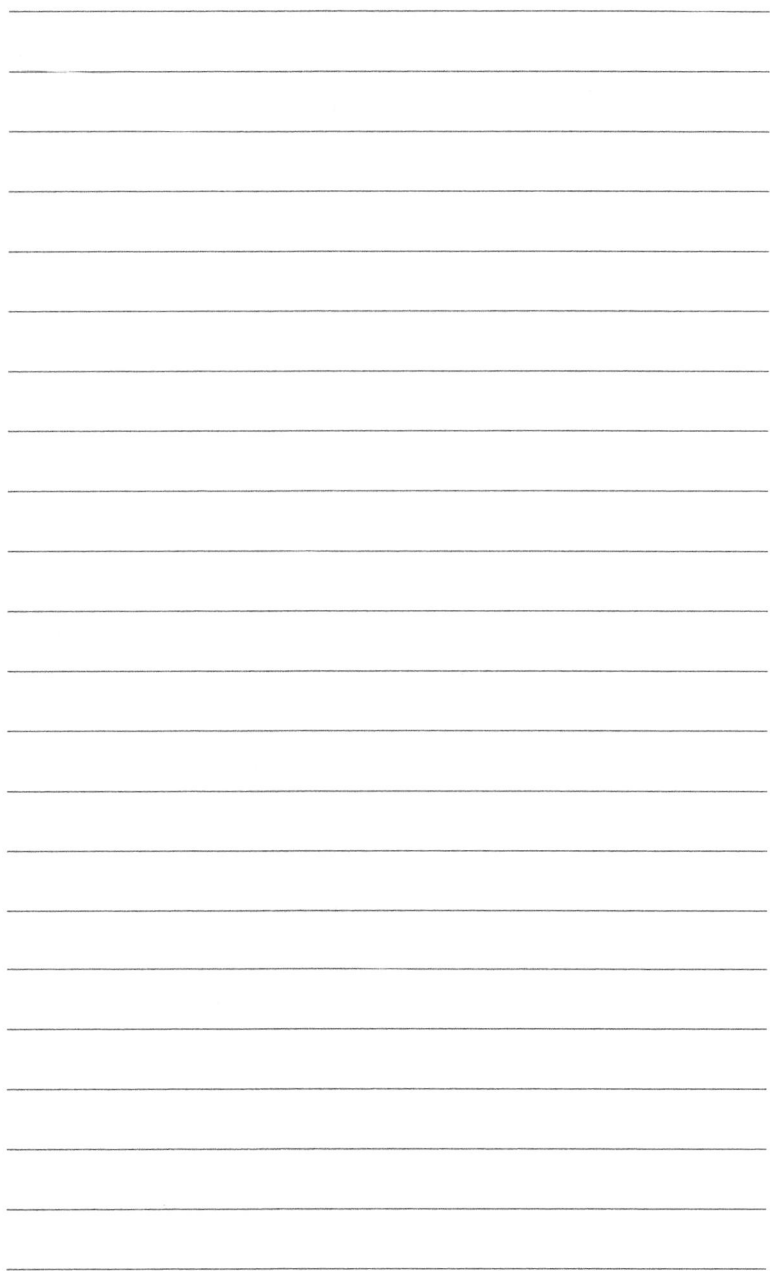

Chapter 12
Social support and Group Programs

> The best part of my job is to see the positive transformation that happens after men feel supported and heard. — Sam Hughes

> Call it a clan, call it a network, call it a tribe, call it a family. Whatever you call it, whoever you are, you need one. — Jane Howard

Social support in cancer care refers to the assistance, comfort, and encouragement provided by family members, friends, support groups, healthcare professionals, and other individuals or organizations to individuals diagnosed with cancer and their loved ones.

Social support and integration serve as a milestone for health and happiness, and have been linked to improved emotional health, quality of life, and even reduced morbidity and mortality in cancer patients. (21) (22)

Social support can take on diverse forms, such as:

- Receiving emotional encouragement from partners and family members
- Gaining access to valuable information
- Engaging in peer groups and gatherings
- Participating in structured sessions
- Joining group activities that cultivate a sense of commonality among individuals

Isolation can be be a prevalent issue among prostate cancer survivors, as they may find themselves withdrawing and enduring their struggles alone, potentially hindering their healing process.

Finding a safe and trusting space to allow men to share similar experiences and problems can be very beneficial during the recovery process.

It's important to actively seek support from various sources such as family, friends, support groups, or by becoming involved in a prostate cancer support system. Engaging with a prostate cancer support group can facilitate deeper connections with local resources and fellow individuals navigating similar challenges.

Additionally, the guidance of prostate cancer group facilitators can be invaluable, offering both support and a wealth of knowledge.

GROUP FITNESS PROGRAMS

An effective approach to promoting social integration and other health-related benefits is to encourage prostate cancer survivors to join a group fitness program. Some men may find themselves more motivated to participate in an 'action-oriented' program, such as a fitness exercise class, rather than talk-based programs. These exercise programs not only provide a space for physical activity but also foster emotional connections and facilitate information sharing, contributing to improvements in both physical and mental health.

A note from the author:

When I started working with prostate cancer clients, I wanted to test if they would do well in a group program (as my waitlist was increasing). I ran a small study to identify if the same intervention (treatment) would be effective if administered in a group setting. The results were encouraging - all participants had positive feedback about the group program. Their feedback was how they felt the support they received from others helped them in the healing process. As well as mood change, their incontinence episodes improved after 8 weeks of the program and continued to improve for 6 months.

Once I concluded the research, I developed a program to encourage the prostate surgical patients to attend a group session prior to seeing the pelvic floor physical therapists one-on-one. This allowed them to receive the educational material as soon as possible, but also gave them the opportunity to interact with each other. I collected data for several years from post-evaluation questionnaires, and the results were suggestive of a well-received and successful program. Since then I've been continuing to stress the importance of seeing this population in a group format.

Notes

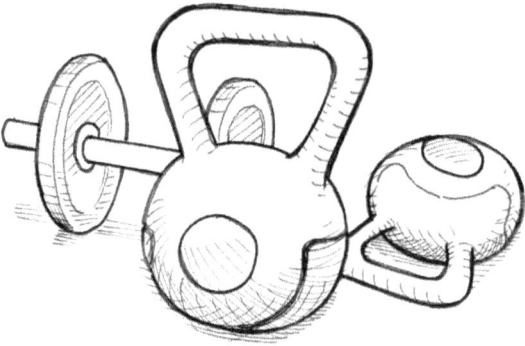

Chapter 13
Exercise

It is recommended for most prostate cancer patients to exercise regularly. Regular physical activity (which includes a combination of resistance and aerobic training) can improve muscular strength, aerobic endurance, muscle mass, functional performance, as well as overall health and quality of life (23). Physical activity may slow prostate cancer progression (24) (25).

Aerobics:

Aerobic exercise gets the heart rate up, and includes exercises such as walking, stair climbing, running, cycling, and swimming. It is recommended to perform at least 2.5 to 3 hours of aerobic exercise per week. The heart rate should measure in between 60 to 80% of your maximum heart rate, and those who have cardiac conditions should consult with their health care provider for personalized guidelines. Aerobic exercises can also help maintain body weight, which can therefore reduce chances of developing diabetes, cardiac diseases, and can help reduce urinary incontinence by reducing intra-abdominal pressure.

Walking programs are the safest form of aerobics, especially right after surgery. The benefits of aerobic exercises are usually experienced after 20-30 minutes of consistent optimal heart rate at least 2-3 times a week.

Strength training:

Strength training improves muscle tone, fights muscle loss and helps to maintain bone density. It can be done with exercise machines, dumbbells, weighted elastics, or barbells. Weight training can also be done by using the body as a form of weight: exercises such as planks, push-ups, sit-ups, squats, lunges, and bridging. Strength training should be done at least twice a week for maintaining muscle mass, especially in the older population [23].

It is important to listen to the body to identify how much weight to use to avoid injuries and pain. The safest weight training program is to use less weight and more repetitions. Posture and good body mechanics should be used to avoid injury and to improve muscle coordination and contraction. If pain is limiting exercise tolerance, modify the exercises or consult with an exercise specialist or physical therapist before continuing.

Stretching:

Muscle shortening due to poor posture or certain activities may be a risk for future injuries. Stretching should be part of the exercise routine to improve muscle length and coordination. Stretching should be done after strength training. Improving muscle length (especially in the lower body), can help with pelvic floor muscle dysfunction, especially in men who have difficulties with relaxation. Stretching should be done on a regular basis, holding the posture for a few minutes at a time without provoking pain. For a more successful stretching routine, the stretching sensation should be minimal in order to allow muscles to effectively relax and progressively change length.

Case 3:

A client that went through one of my group education classes was seen for a follow-up one year later. I didn't recognise him, as he was probably 50 pounds lighter and very fit. After learning all the benefits of weight management and health, he decided to work with a personal trainer to help improve his strength and to lose weight. One year later he was lean and strong and much happier with his life. He was running 5-6 km, 3-4 times a week and reported that running was helping him maintain dryness as well as controlling his anxiety and depression. He was so inspired by his recovery process that he became involved in sharing his experience with others, motivating and inspiring men after prostate cancer surgery.

How to calculate maximum heart rate

Maximum heart rate or MHR is calculated by subtracting your age from 220.

For example, for a 65 year-old male, his maximum heart rate should be 155 beats per minute (220-65=155).

In order for him to exercise at 80% MHR, his targeted heart rate should be 124 BPM.

Consult with your physician or health care provider prior to exercising, especially if it is new to you or if undergoing chemotherapy or radiation.

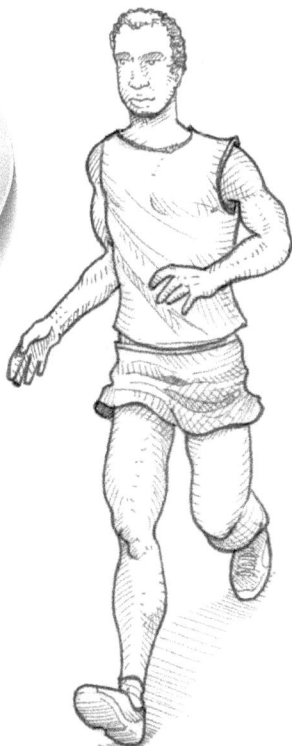

Notes

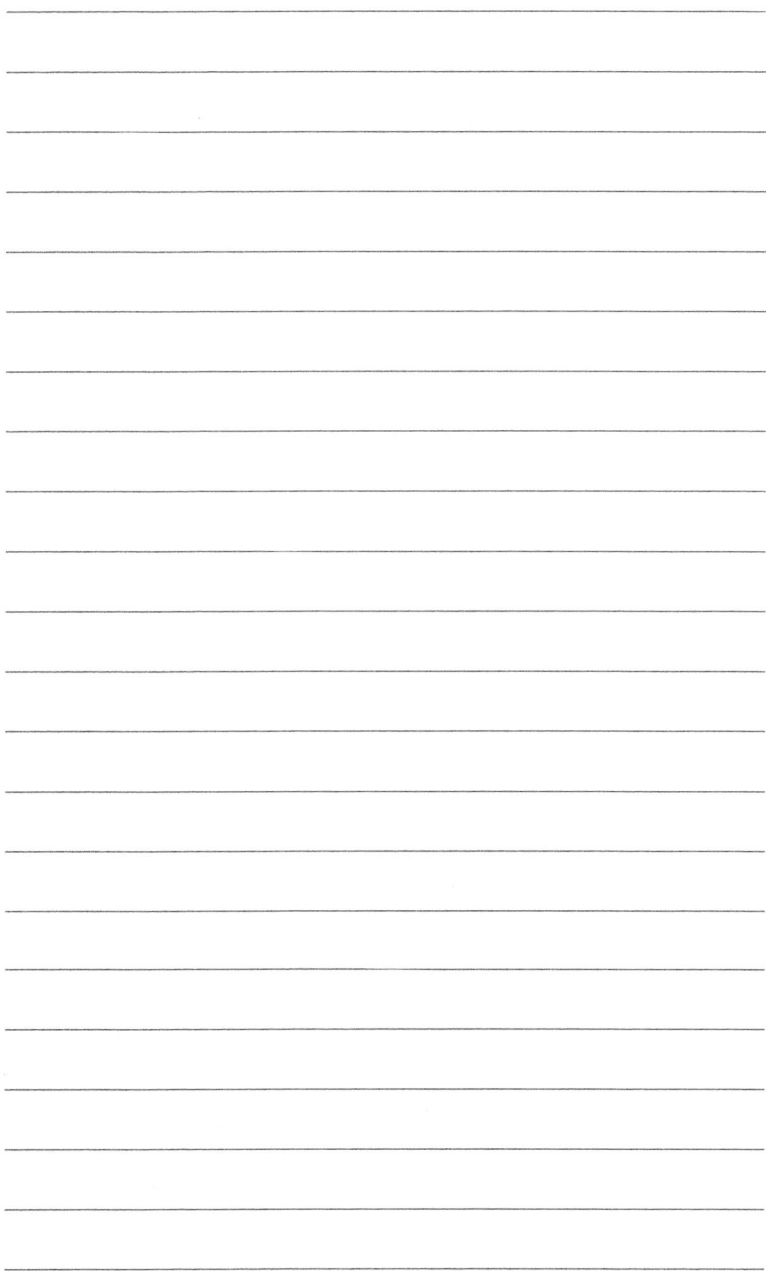

Chapter 14
Final thoughts

In summary, there are many factors which could influence and affect men's recovery after prostate surgery. Understanding the surgery and the cause of its side effects can be valuable to improve men's confidence and outcome.

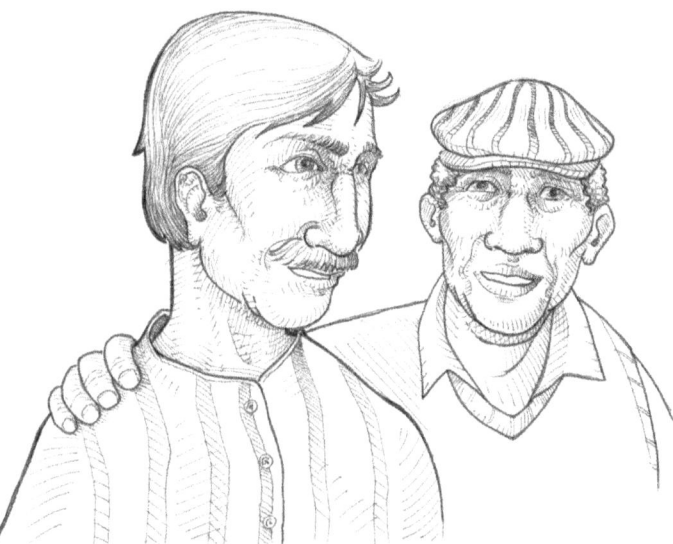

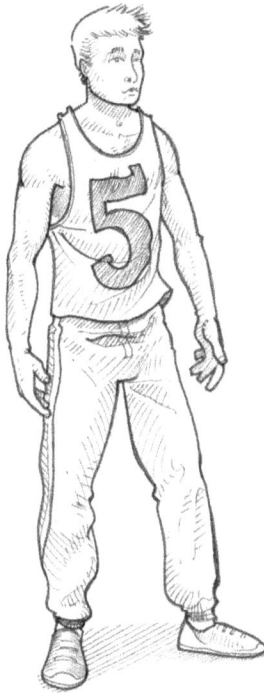

Treating the body holistically and managing factors which influence recovery is the key for improvement. The bladder and sexual function can recuperate faster with healthy drinking and eating habits, regular bowel routines, taking care of mental health, performing appropriate pelvic floor exercises, increasing physical activity, and having a support system. The optimal goal is to live a healthy and positive life and manage the potential side-effects of prostate cancer surgery in the best way possible.

Notes

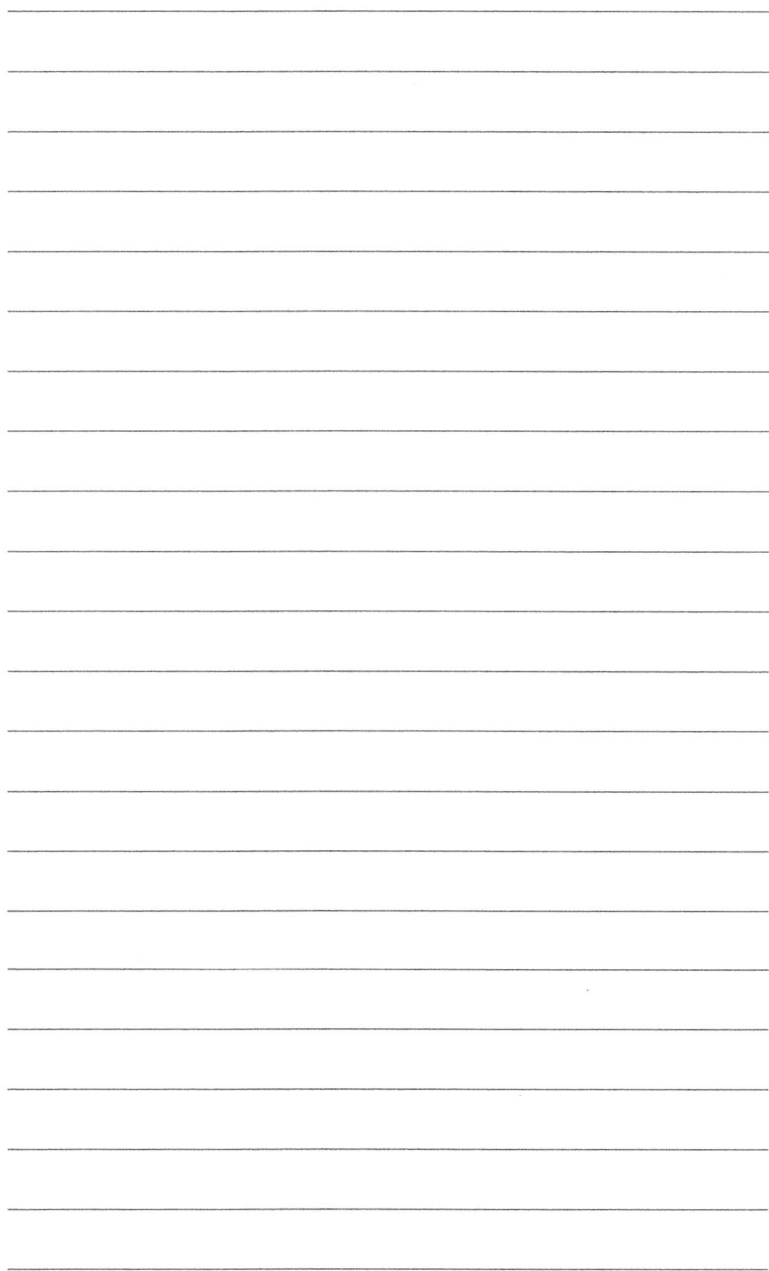

1. Global cancer statistics 2018: GLOBOCAN estimates of incidence and mortality worldwide for 36 cancers in 185 countries. Bray F, Ferlay J, Soerjomataram I, Siegel RL, Torre LA & Jemal A. CA: A Cancer Journal for Clinicians, 2018, Vol. 68.

2. International Variation in Prostate Cancer Incidence and Mortality Rates. Center MM, Jemal A, Lortet-Tieulent J, Ward E, Ferlay J, Brawley O & Bray F. European Urology, Vol. 61. 1079-1092.

3. Cancer treatment and survivorship statistics, 2014. DeSantis CE, Lin CC, Mariotto AB, Siegel RL, Stein KD, Kramer JL, Alteri R, Robbins AS & Jemal A. CA, 2014, Vol. 64. 252-271.

4. Urinary incontinence in men. Bauer RM, Oelke M, Hübner W, Grabbert M, Kirschner-Hermanns R & Anding R. Urologe A., 2015, Vol. 54. 887-99.

5. Review of the comparative effectiveness of radical prostatectomy, radiation therapy, or expectant management of localized prostate cancer in registry data. Serrell EC, Pitts D, Hayn M, Beaule L, Hansen MH & Sammon JD. Urologic Oncology, 2018, Vol. 36. 183-192.

6. The pathophysiology of post-radical prostatectomy incontinence: a clinical and video urodynamic study. Groutz A, Blaivas JG, Chaikin DC, Weiss JP & Verhaaren M. The Journal of Urology, 2000, Vol. 163. 1767-1770.

7. Treatment options for male stress urinary incontinence. Sandhu, JS. Nature Reviews Urology, 2010, Vol. 7. 222-228.

8. Post-radical prostatectomy incontinence: Etiology and prevention. Hoyland K et al. Reviews in Urology, 16(4) 181-188

9. Urinary incontinence and quality of life among older community-dwelling Australian men: the CHAMP study. Kwong PW, Cumming RG, Chan L, Seibel MJ, Naganathan V, Creasey H, Le Couteur D, Waite LM, Sambrook PN & Handelsman D. Age and Ageing, 2010, Vol. 39. 349-354.

10. Behavioral Therapy With or Without Biofeedback and Pelvic Floor Electrical Stimulation for Persistent Postprostatectomy Incontinence. Goode PS, Burgio KL, Johnson TM 2nd, Clay OJ, Roth DL, Markland AD, Burkhardt JH, Issa MM & Lloyd LK. JAMA, 2011, Vol. 305. 151-59.

11. Pelvic floor muscle trainning in radical prostatectomy. A randomized control trial of the impacts on pelvic floor muscle function and urinary incontinence. Milios JE. et al. BMC Urology Vol. 19 (1). 116.

12. Recognition and Management of Nonrelaxing Pelvic Floor Dysfunction. Faubion SS, Shuster LT & Bharucha AE. Mayo Clinic Proceedings, 2012, Vol. 87. 187-193.

13. The Association of Depressive Symptoms and Urinary Incontinence Among Older Adults. Dugan E, Cohen SJ, Bland DR, Preisser JS, Davis CC, Suggs PK & McGann P. Journal of American Geriatrics Society, 2000, Vol. 48. 357-466.

14. Understanding the stress response. Harvard Health Publishing Harvard Medical School. [Online] March 2011. https://www.health.harvard.edu/staying-healthy understanding-the-stress-response.

15. Erectile dysfunction following prostatectomy: prevention and treatment. Magheli A, & Burnett AL. Nature Reviews Urology, 2009, Vol. 6. 415-27.

16. Factors Predicting Recovery of Erections after Radical Prostatectomy. Rabbani F, Stapleton AM, Kattan MW, Wheeler TM & Scardino PT. Journal of Urology, 2000, Vol. 164. 1929-1934.

17. Penile rehabilitation for post prostatectomy erectile dysfunction: A Cochrane Systematic Review and Meta-analysis. Philippou YA, Jung J, Steggall MJ, O'Driscoll ST, Bakker CJ, Bodie JA & Dahm P. The Journal of Urology, 2018, Vol. 199. e1172.

18. Recovery of spontaneous erectile function after nerve-sparing radical retropubic prostatectomy with and without early intracavernous injections of alprostadil: results of a prospective, randomized trial. Montorsi et al. J Urol ,1997, Vol. 158 (4) 1408-10.

19. Sexuality Following Radical Prostatectomy: Is Restoration of Erectile Function Enough? Fode M, Serefoglu EC, Albersen M & Sønksen J. Sexual Medicine Reviews, 2017, Vol. 5. 110-119.

20. Pelvic floor muscle training for erectile dysfunction and climacturia 1 year after nerve sparing radical prostatectomy: a randomized controlled trial. Geraerts I, Van Poppel H, Devoogdt N, De Groef A, Fieuws S & Van Kampen M. International Journal of Impotence Research, 2016, Vol. 28. 9-13.

21. The effects of social support on health-related quality of life of patients with metastatic prostate cancer. Collaca, G & Colloca P. Journal of Cancer Education, 2019, Vol 31 (2), 244-252.

22. Effects of social support, hope and resilience on depressive symptoms within 18 months after diagnosis of prostate cancer. Zhao et al. Health and Quality of Life Outcome, 2021. Vol 19(1), 15.

21. Body Composition, Physical Fitness, Functional Performance, Quality of Life, and Fatigue Benefits of Exercise for Prostate Cancer Patients: A Systematic Review. RD, Keogh JWL & MacLeod. Journal of Pain and Symptom Management, 2012, Vol. 43. 96-110.

22. Physical Activity and Survival After Prostate Cancer Diagnosis in the Health Professionals Follow-Up Study. Kenfield SA, Stampfer MJ, Giovannucci E & Chan JM. Clinical Oncology, Vol. 29. 726-732.

23. Physical Activity after Diagnosis and Risk of Prostate Cancer Progression: Data from the Cancer of the Prostate Strategic Urologic Research Endeavor. Richman EL, Kenfield SA, Stampfer MJ, Paciorek A, Carroll PR & Chan JM. Cancer Research, 2011, Vol. 71. 1-7.

23. The benefits of strength training for older adults. ME, Seguin R & Nelson. American Journal of Preventive Medicine, 2003, Vol. 25. 141-149.

Herman Kwan,
B.Sc. Pharm., MD, FRCSC
– Urologist

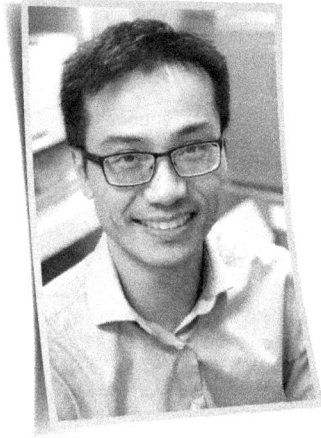

Dr. Kwan was born in Vancouver, Canada and spend his childhood in White Rock, Canada. He completed a pharmacy degree and then a medical degree at the University of British Columbia (UBC) in Canada. He completed a Urology residency at UBC and a fellowship in laparoscopy and robotics at the Swedish Medical Centre in Seattle under Dr James Porter. He is interested in Radical Prostatectomy, especially in high risk disease setting and nerve sparing approaches. He currently works in White Rock, Canada.

Question 1: I had my surgery 1 month ago. I feel I have no urinary control and need to wear many pull-ups a day. I feel frustrated and sad about the slow progress, and I wonder if I am ever going to improve?

Answer 1: During the first few months after the surgery urinary incontinence can be significant because it is the period where the body is still recovering. Normally urinary incontinence will improve, and many men can be dry after 6 to 12 months after surgery.

Question 2: What predicts the return of urinary continence after the surgery?

Answer 2: It is quite unpredictable how a man will recover his urinary control. The outcome of the surgery doesn't seem to be a predictor of urinary control — there are men who can be dry at 6-8 weeks, yet others only start to recover after 6 months post surgery. Generally speaking younger men will recover faster than older men (over 70 years of age).

Question 3: My surgeon did not perform nerve sparing surgery. Will this affect urinary recovery?

Answer 3: Nerve sparing surgery, usually performed for preservation of erectile function, may not be a predictor for urinary control. Some people believe that after a nerve sparing procedure there may be better urinary control, however this has not yet been proven in studies. In my experience, when we do non-sparing surgery, lots of those patients regain very good urinary control.

Question 4: When can I start exercising after the surgery?

Answer 4: After surgery we encourage patients to start walking right away. The main thing is to listen to your body, as long as you are not in any discomfort, you can walk and climb stairs as you wish. However, you should not lift more than 20 lb, for 6 weeks post surgery. After the 6 weeks you can progress as tolerated.

Question 5: My penis seems smaller after the surgery, is this normal?

Answer 5: This is a very common observation for many patients. Most Urologists think it is because of some large vessels of the penis being ligated (tied together), which decreases the blood flow to the penis and can cause penile atrophy.

Dr. Dinesh Samarasekera,
MD, FRCSC – Urologist

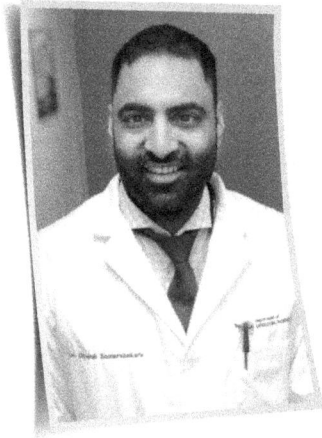

Dr. Samarasekera's medical degree was obtained from the University of British Columbia in 2007. He completed his residency in Urology at UBC, obtaining his fellowship (FRCSC) in 2012. After a two-year fellowship in robotic and laparoscopic surgery at the Cleveland Clinic in Ohio, Dr. Samarasekera returned to Vancouver. He also holds a degree in mechanical engineering.

Dr. Samarasekera's urological practice is based out of Surrey, BC, Canada.

Question 6: How soon can I begin penile rehabilitation after surgery?

Answer 6: Men can begin penile rehabilitation as soon as the catheter comes out after surgery. It typically involves taking a PDE5 inhibitor (ie. Cialis, Viagra, Levitra) a few times a week to stimulate blood flow.

Question 7: What are the most common treatments for erectile dysfunction?

Answer 7: The common treatments for erectile dysfunction are:

a.) Medications – Sildenafil (Viagra) Tadalafil (Cialis) Vardenafil (Levitra)

b.) A vacuum pump device

c.) Cavernosal Injections (Trimix – phentolamine, alprostadil, papaverine)

d.) Implantable penile prosthesis (malleable or inflatable – AMS)

Question 8: Can I still achieve orgasm without an erection?

Answer 8: The simple answer is yes you can. The sensation will be much the same as it was before, but the orgasm will now be a dry orgasm. You will have no ejaculate fluid coming out after the surgery because during the surgery the vas deferens is disconnected and the seminal vesicles removed (these are where all the fluid comes from).

During an orgasm the nerves that go to the head of the penis and send messages to the brain promotes the perception of sexual stimuli. This process is independent of the ejaculation and erection, so it can work independently. Nerves are still working on sending messages to the brain but because the plumbing [so to speak] is disconnected, you still have the orgasm but without the ejaculation.

Occasionally, men can experience some urinary leakage during orgasm after prostate removal surgery.

Question 9: I had my Prostate removed but my PSA level seems to be slowly rising. What does that mean, and what should I do?

Answer 9: A rising PSA after radical prostatectomy could mean a number of different things. One possibility is that there could be some residual benign prostate tissue left over. The other possibility is recurrent cancer. The most important thing is to follow up with your urologist who will do a physical examination and possible imaging such as an MRI or CT scan and sometimes a biopsy of the place where the prostate was. If it continues to rise it may be evidence of recurrent cancer and you may need radiation therapy or Androgen deprivation therapy (Hormonal Therapy).

Question 10: When should I consider surgery to treat urinary incontinence after prostate cancer surgery? What type of surgery and how effective is it?

Answer 10: I usually council men to consider surgery after prostate cancer surgery to correct incontinence if there is no significant improvement in urinary incontinence after at least a year – and this includes having tried physical therapy.

Usually surgery is recommended when men are having ongoing leakages, requiring pads and the symptoms are bothersome for them. Options include either a urethral sling surgery or artificial sphincter implant. The surgery is dependent on the degree of incontinence that you have. If you have mild incontinence the sling can be effective, but if the incontinence is more severe the artificial urinary sphincter would be the surgery of choice. Both procedures are highly effective if done properly and most men can be significantly dry afterwards.

With the sling most men should have a durable long-term result (at least 10 years or longer) if done correctly and the incontinence is mild. With regards to the Artificial Urinary Sphincter Surgery men could have a long-term success rate but there is a greater risk of infection or a loss of urethral pressure over time. Most men do very well with the surgery and have a good long-term success.

Appendix 1
Urinary Urgency

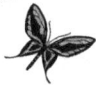

Information provided by BC Women's Hospital Continence Clinic 2016

How to Control Urinary Urgency

Every time you feel the urge to urinate, stop immediately and get control. Settle every urge before walking to the bathroom.

The following tips will help you to settle the urge:

- **If you are walking:** stop moving!!

- **If you are standing:** sit if possible.

- **Tighten up your pelvic floor muscles** (if indicated). You can also do a few mini pumps with your muscles. Repeat 2 to 6 times and then hold again, depending on the strength of the urge. Visualize how your muscles are clamping around your urethra, the tube leading from the bladder.

- **Use positive self-talk.** Tell your bladder to "Stop it!" Tell it to calm down. Tell yourself "I will not leak"! Believe you can get control! Remember YOU are the boss, not your bladder.

- **Stay calm. Breathe.** Tell yourself "I will not let a drop out. I am in control."

- **Distraction improves control.**

- **Try rubbing the back of your thighs a few times**, curling your toes or rising up on the balls of your feet to calm your bladder. These will have a calming effect and help settle the urge.

- **At home press your hand against the area where the urine comes out.** This calms your bladder and reduces urgency.

Be aware of triggers that may cause a strong urge:

- **"Key in the door"**- as you arrive home*
- **Running water**
- **Seeing the toilet**
- **Freezer aisle of the supermarket**
- **Cold, wet weather**

To settle these, tighten up your pelvic floor muscles - do a few short hold'ems, talk to your bladder, don't move, wait for the urge to pass before moving. It will!

*With "key in the door" problem, empty your bladder before going home. When you get home, settle the urge using urge control techniques. Then do a few things around the house like turning on the kettle, or your computer, check phone messages etc.

Do not go immediately to the bathroom. You are trying to break the habit of coming home and running to the bathroom.

Tips to Reduce Urinary Urgency

- **Bladder irritants:** Avoid or reduce foods/drinks that irritate your bladder.

- **Constipation:** Avoid it.

- **Strengthen your pelvic floor muscles.**
  They will hold the urine better and they will calm your bladder more effectively.

- **Fluids:** Don't restrict them. Drink at least 5 cups of fluid per day. Water is best. Spread your fluids through the day, and limit fluids in the evening. Don't drink too much fluid!

- **Use the toilet at regular intervals in the daytime.**
  Ideally you want to urinate every 2-4 hours. Don't wait longer. If you urinate more often, ask yourself, "Could I wait 5 minutes longer?" Try to delay urinating just for a few minutes, if you can.

- **See your family doctor and get your urine checked if urgency is a problem.** You want to make sure you don't have an infection.

- See your family doctor if there is **blood in your urine.**

Appendix 2

How to manage constipation

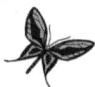

Information provided by BC Women's Hospital Continence Clinic 2016

FIBER

HOW MUCH DO YOU REALLY NEED?

• You need 25 to 35 grams of fiber a day. Ideally you want to eat a mixture of soluble and insoluble fiber (more on that later).

• Try to eat a diet that is high in fiber and low in saturated fats.

Avoid processed and fast foods.

YOUR DRINKS

• Drink 6-8 cups of fluid per day. Drinking an adequate amount of fluid will help to keep your bowels regular.

- When the weather is hot and after exercise you will need to drink more.

- Fill a water bottle in the morning and sip on it through the day. If you are going out take it with you. Refill as it runs out. Avoid fluids in the evening.

YOUR EXERCISE

- Exercise several times per week helps to keep bowel movements regular. Choose some form of exercise that you enjoy and that you can realistically fit into your daily routine. Consider a daily walk and some abdominal exercises.

- Look for ways to be more active. For example, take the stairs rather than the elevator, park your car at the far end of the parking lot rather than close to the door, or get off the bus a few blocks before your stop.

- Your physical therapist can give you exercise ideas.

- If you have any health problems consult your family doctor before starting an exercise program to ensure the program is suitable for you.

YOUR BOWELS

- Try to empty your bowels at the same time each day.

- The bowels tend to become active after you eat. Try to have your bowel movements after a meal. If the best time is after breakfast, then make sure you get up early enough so you have time.

- If you tend to be constipated, eat insoluble fiber (fibrous vegetables) which increases stool bulk, making the stool softer and speeds up the time it takes to move the stool through the intestines.

Examples of insoluble fiber:

- Whole grains, wheat bran, most beans, lentils, dried fruits and fibrous vegetables with edible skins and seeds, corn, popcorn.

If you have a tendency to have loose stools you might have a sensitivity or allergy to some foods. The most common foods causing this are tomatoes, nuts, milk, caffeine, alcohol, spices and sugar substitutes, especially Sorbitol, Zolotol, and Saccharin. Soluble fiber helps form gel in the stool making it more formed.

Examples of soluble fiber:

- Psyllium (Metamucil), oatmeal, barley, rye, beans such as kidney, garbanzo, lentils and split peas, oranges, fruits including apples and pears.

- Excessive caffeine intake should be avoided. If you feel you have food sensitivities, you should see a registered dietitian for proper management.

Soluble fibre helps to:

- Lower blood cholesterol levels. Aim for at least 10 grams of soluble fibre every day.

- Control blood glucose (sugar) levels. This is helpful if you have diabetes or if you sometimes get a low blood sugar (hypoglycaemia)

- Manage diarrhea and loose stools

- Reduce some of the symptoms of Irritable Bowel Syndrome

- Reduce the risk of getting intestinal ulcers

- Have a healthier colon by increasing the amount of healthy bacteria.

GOOD SOURCES OF FIBRE

The following fibre sources are especially ranked for fibre content. The A category is the highest, with over 7 g per serving. B is next with three or more periods and see foods have less than 3 g.

The list of high fibre foods below can help you reduce your risk of constipation, hemorrhoids, high cholesterol, high blood sugar, obesity, Colon cancer, diabetes and heart disease.

Most people only get about 10 g of fibre a day. That's not nearly enough. You need 25 to 35 g of fibre a day for optimum health.

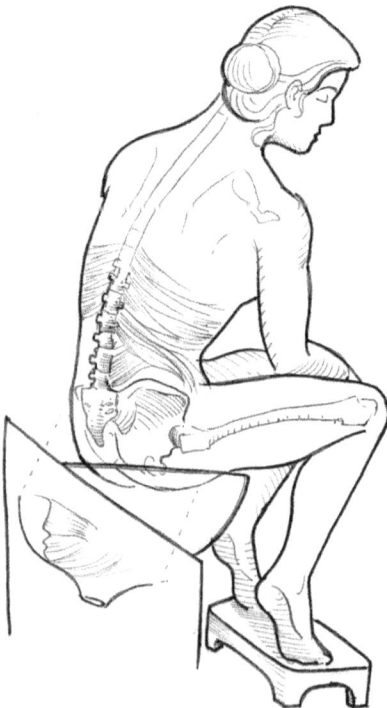

Please use the following list to assist you.

HIGH-FIBER FOOD CHART

Category A (more than 7 g per serving)

FOOD	AMOUNT	TOTAL FIBER (grams)
Avocado	1 medium	11.84
Barley	1/2 cup	15
Black beans, cooked	1 cup	14.92
Bran cereal	1 cup	19.94
Broccoli, cooked	1 cup	4.50
Green peas, cooked	1 cup	8.84
Kale, cooked	1 cup	7.20
Kidney beans, cooked	1 cup	13.33
Lentils, cooked	1 cup	15.64
Lima beans, cooked	1 cup	13.16
Navy beans, cooked	1 cup	11.65
Oats, dry	1 cup	12
Pinto beans, cooked	1 cup	14.71
Split peas, cooked	1 cup	16.27
Raspberries	1 cup	8.34
Rice, brown, uncooked	1 cup	7.98
Soybeans, cooked	1 cup	7.62

(The fiber count for most packaged foods can be found on the label.)

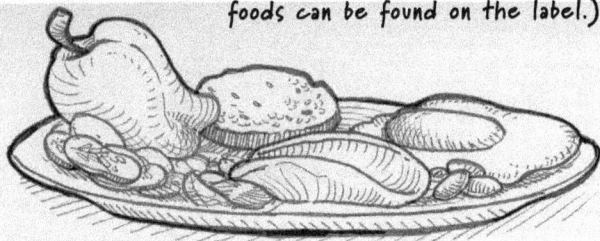

Category B (more than 3 grams per serving)

FOOD	AMOUNT	TOTAL FIBER (grams)
Almonds	1 oz.	4.22
Apple, w/ skin	1 medium	5.00
Banana	1 medium	3.92
Blueberries	1 cup	4.18
Cabbage, cooked	1 cup	4.20
Cauliflower	1 cup	3.43
Corn, sweet	1 cup	4.66
Figs, dried	2 medium	3.74
Flax seeds	3 tsp.	6.97
Garbanzo beans, cooked	1 cup	5.80
Grapefruit	1/2 medium	6.12
Green beans, cooked	1 cup	3.95
Olives	1 cup	4.30
Orange, navel	1 medium	3.40
Papaya	1 each	5.47
Pasta, whole wheat	1 cup	6.34
Peach, dried	3 pcs.	3.18
Pear with skin	1 medium	5.08
Pistachio nuts	1 oz.	3.10
Potato, baked w/ skin	medium	4.80
Prunes	1/4 cup	3.02
Pumpkin seeds	1/4 cup	4.12
Sesame seeds	1/4 cup	4.32
Strawberries	1 cup	3
Sweet potato, cooked	1 cup	3.68
Swiss chard, cooked	1 cup	5.04
Wheat germ	1 oz.	4.05
Winter Squash	1 cup	5.74
Yam, cooked cubes	1 cup	5.30

Category C (less than 3 g per serving)

FOOD	AMOUNT	TOTAL FIBER (grams)
Apricots	3 medium	0.98
Apricots, dried	5 pieces	2.89
Asparagus, cooked	1 cup	2.88
Beets, cooked	1 cup	2.85
Bread: whole wheat	1 slice	2.00
Brussels sprouts, cooked	1 cup	2.84
Cantaloupe	1 cup	1.28
Carrots, raw	1 medium	2.00
Cashews	1 oz.	1.00
Celery	1 stalk	1.00
Cherries	1/2 cup	0.56
Collard greens, cooked	1 cup	2.58
Cranberries	1/2 cup	1.99
Cucumber, sliced w/ peel	1 cup	0.83
Eggplant, cooked cubes	1 cup	2.48
Grapes	1/2 cup	0.56
Kiwi fruit	1 each	2.58
Mushroom, raw	1 cup	1.36
Mustard greens, cooked	1 cup	2.80
Onions, raw	1 cup	2.88
Peanuts	1 oz.	2.30
Peach	1 medium	2.00
Peppers, sweet	1 cup	2.62
Plum	1 medium	1.00
Popcorn (pooped)	1/2 cup	0.53
Raisins	1.5 oz box	1.60
Rice (white)	1/2 cup	1.42
Romaine lettuce	1 cup	0.95
Summer squash, cooked	1 cup	2.52
Sunflower seeds	1/4 cup	3.00
Tomato	1 medium	1.00
Walnuts	1 oz.	2.98
Wax beans (yellow)	1 cup	3.78
Zucchini, cooked	1 cup	2.63

Appendix 3
Diaphragmatic Breathing

Diaphragmatic Breathing strengthens the diaphragm muscles (domed shaped muscles at the base of the lungs). Once the diaphragm is used correctly through deep breathing, it can decrease the work of breathing while promoting relaxation

There is a close relationship between the diaphragm and the pelvic floor muscles. During normal respiration, or any event of diaphragmatic change (such as coughing), a change in the pelvic floor muscles is observed. For example, during inspiration the diaphragm muscles and the pelvic floor muscles will descend simultaneously. [1]

Diaphragmatic breathing technique

1. Lie comfortably on your back with knees supported under a pillow. Spend a few minutes focusing on your breathing. Place one hand on your chest and the other hand over your lower abdomen. Try to slow down your breathing by increasing your expiration time. You can even count slowly to 2 when you inhale and to 4 when your exhale. Inhale through your nose and exhale slowly from your mouth. Try not to force expiration, just let the air flow out passively.

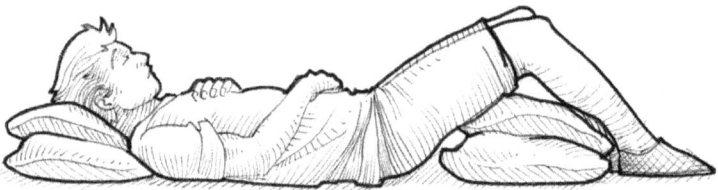

Once you master this breathing technique in a lying position, you can try diaphragmatic breathing in a sitting position, or in any of the opening postures shown below (Appendix 4). Visualize pelvic floor muscle relaxation especially during inspiration. This breathing strategy can also help with pelvic floor muscle relaxation and pelvic pain.

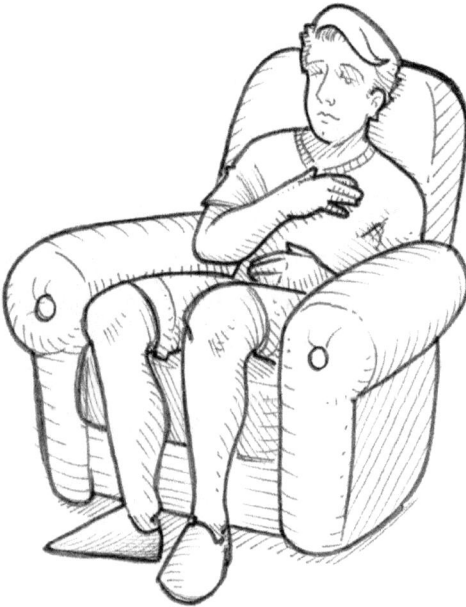

1. Phase-locked parallel movement of diaphragm and pelvic floor during breathing and coughing-a dynamic MRI investigation in healthy females. Talasz H, Kremser C, Kofler M, Kalchschmid E, Lechleitner M & Rudisch A. 1, s.l. : Int Urogynecol J., 2011, Vol. 22. 61-68.

2. Visualize the hand over your upper chest being heavier than the hand over your lower abdomen. Inhale through your nose allowing your lower abdomen to rise, without moving your upper chest. Visualize a balloon being inflated right underneath your lower abdomen.

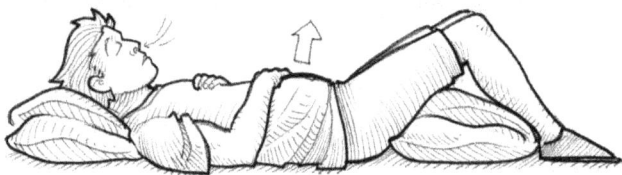

3. Exhale, slowly out your mouth, letting the air fall from your lower abdomen without pushing the air out or contracting the abdominal muscles.

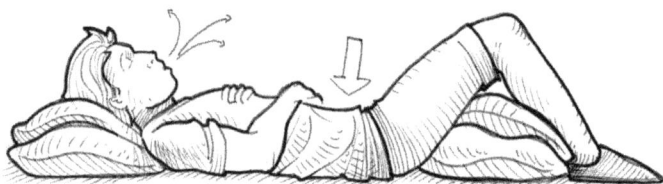

4. Continue to inhale and exhale, noticing your abdomen rising and falling, making sure your upper chest remains quiet. Practice this breathing for 5–10 minutes, 3 times a day.

Appendix 4
Opening Stretches

Example of opening poses

Stay in these poses 2 to 5 min at the time. The poses should feel comfortable, and the stretching sensation not too intense. Don't over stretch! No pain should be experienced. If the sensation is too intense, modify!

Pose 1:

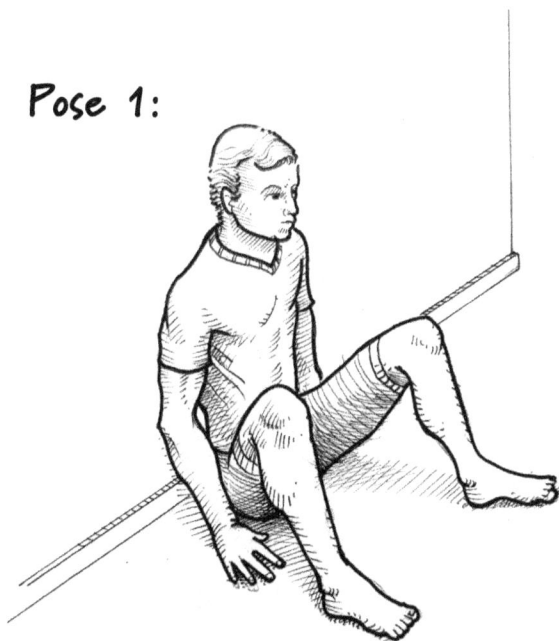

Perineal Stretch

Pose 2:

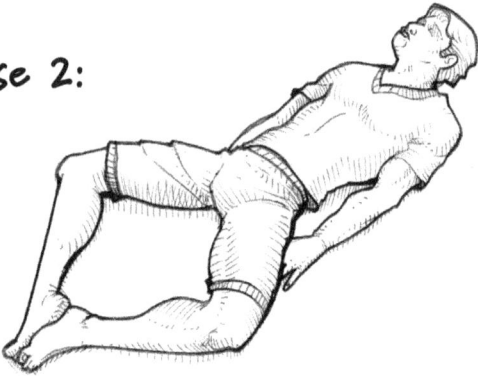

Symmetry Posture

Pose 3:

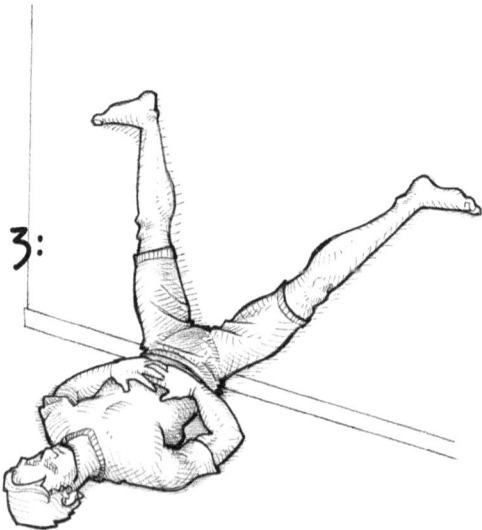

Long adductors Stretch

Pose 4:

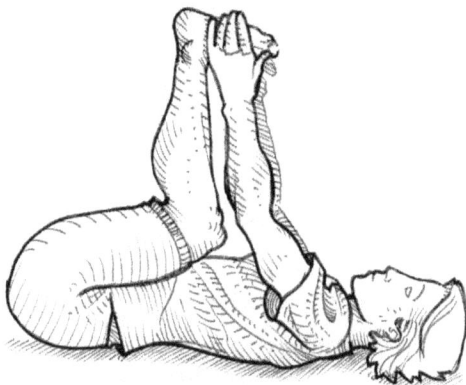

Happy Baby Pose

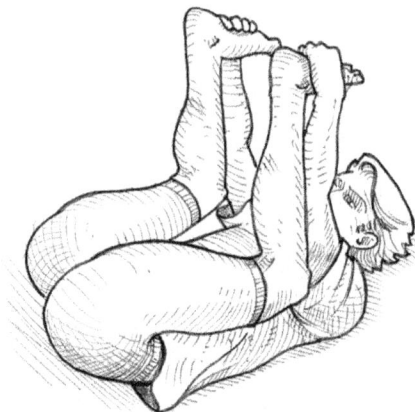

Appendix 5
Healthy Bladder Habits

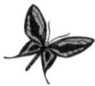

Information provided by BC Women's Hospital Continence Clinic 2016

Keeping a bladder diary can help to be more aware of your bladder habits.

HOW MUCH SHOULD I DRINK?

- You need 1 to 2 liters of fluid every day. This includes all fluids you drink, even soup.

- If you have been exercising and sweating, have an extra cup of water to replace the fluid you have lost.

- Limit the amount of coffee, tea and alcohol you drink. These drinks have a diuretic effect and will tend to "go right through you," causing you to lose fluids rapidly.

WHAT SHOULD I DRINK?

- If you have a problem controlling urinary urgency then avoid drinks that irritate the bladder, such as coffee, alcohol, caffeinated pop, carbonated drinks and strong tea. See the handout, "Bladder Irritants" for a complete list of foods and drinks that cause urinary urgency. Reducing your intake of these fluids will help you to control urgency.

- Water is the best drink. It will not irritate your bladder. Try to drink water instead of other drinks.

WHEN SHOULD I DRINK?

- Spread your fluids throughout the day and sip your fluids, don't gulp down a whole glass at once.

- If you are going out, then take a water bottle with you and sip on it throughout the day. Refill when empty.

- Always have a drink with your meals.

- Drinking after supper might get you up during the night and interrupt your sleep. If this is a problem, then limit your evening fluids and especially any caffeinated beverages.

HOW OFTEN SHOULD I USE THE TOILET?

• In the daytime: emptying your bladder every 2 to 4 hours is considered normal. At night: it is normal to get up once, or if you are over 60 years, twice.

• If you are using the toilet more frequently during the day or night, then speak to a healthcare professional who can help you to regain control.

BLADDER IRRITANTS

Some foods and beverages are known to irritate your bladder. By eliminating or reducing the amount of bladder irritants you drink or eat, you could improve your bladder urgency and the number of times you go to the toilet.

STRONG BLADDER IRRITANTS:

- Caffeine is both a diuretic and bladder irritant. Tea and coffee are equally irritating. After a caffeinated drink, you will produce more urine than the amount of fluid you drank and it will give you a strong urge to go to the toilet. A strong urge might be difficult to control. Some people are also sensitive to decaf coffee or tea.

- Caffeine can also be in medications- check labels on over-the-counter medications and as well as with your pharmacist.

- Carbonated beverages: Bubbly drinks, especially diet pop, are particularly irritating.

- Alcohol is also a diuretic and bladder irritant

**THE FOLLOWING MIGHT IRRITATE
YOUR BLADDER:**

• Certain acidic fruits:
> oranges, grapefruits, lemons and limes,
   strawberries, grapes, peaches, pineapple
   and fruit juices
> cranberry juice (more than 1 cup a day)
> tomato-based products

• Spicy foods, with hot chili peppers

• Chocolate

• Vinegar in large quantity

• Corn syrup

• Cigarettes and all tobacco products

• Vitamins C and B. Try buffered
   vitamin C & B

• Artificial sweeteners eg. Aspartame
   (Equal, Nutrasweet) and Splenda,

Why these items sometimes cause irritation isn't exactly understood, and what causes bladder irritation may vary from person to person.

Most people are not sensitive to ALL of these products, your goal is to find the foods that make YOUR symptoms worse

Water is the best drink

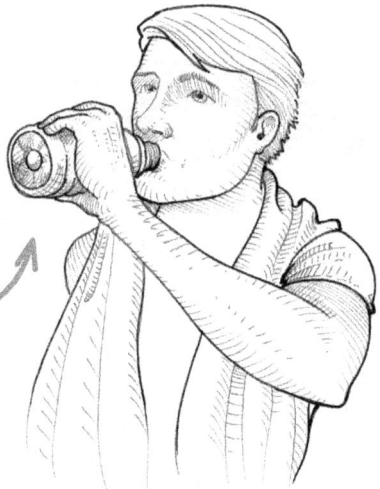

Bladder Diary

How do I keep a 3 day - 24 hour bladder diary?

A bladder diary gives you and your therapist important information about urine leakage and bladder habits. This information helps in planning treatment programs and in evaluating your treatment.

The time that an event happens must always be written in the bladder diary.

When you have a drink, record:
- The time
- The amount (in ozs. or mls)
- What it was you drank.

When you go to the bathroom to empty your bladder:
• Write down the time you went.

When you leak urine write:
• The time
• The amount:
if it was a small, medium, or large amount.
Small = few drops only.
Medium = wet underwear or pad.
Large = soaked clothing or pad.

Finally, write what you think **caused the leakage**. If you experienced a sudden strong urge that caused you to leak, put a tick in the "strong urge" column.

It is best if you keep a bladder diary for 3 consecutive days. To quantify change wait 6-8 weeks before you re do your 3 days - 24 hours bladder diary.

Example: Bladder Diary

Urinary Diary		Day #1	Date: _____		
Time	**Urinated in Toilet**	**Amount and Type of Drink**	**Leakage** Small/Medium/Large	**Reason for Urine Leakage**	**Strong Urge?**
05:30 AM	✓				
07:00 AM		1 c. tea			
08:30 AM	✓				
10:00 AM		1 c. coffee			
11:30 AM			small	walking	✓
01:00 PM	✓				
02:30 PM		1 c. milk			
04:00 PM	✓				
05:30 PM		1 diet cola			
07:00 PM			medium	cough	
08:30 PM	✓				
10:00 PM	✓		small	sneeze	
11:30 PM					
01:00 AM	✓	1 c. water			
03:00 AM	✓				

NOTES: _____ I have a cold, coughing and sneezing more than usual. _____

_____

NUMBER AND TYPE OF PADS USED TODAY: _____ 2 maxi menstrual pads _____

_____

Bladder Diary - 1st set

Urinary Diary	Day#1		Date: _____		
Time	**Urinated in Toilet**	**Amount and Type of Drink**	**Leakage** Small/Medium/Large	**Reason for Urine Leakage**	**Strong Urge?**
05:30 AM					
07:00 AM					
08:30 AM					
10:00 AM					
11:30 AM					
01:00 PM					
02:30 PM					
04:00 PM					
05:30 PM					
07:00 PM					
08:30 PM					
10:00 PM					
11:30 PM					
01:00 AM					
03:00 AM					

NOTES: _____

_____

NUMBER AND TYPE OF PADS USED TODAY: _____

_____

Example: Bladder Diary

Urinary Diary		Day#2	Date: _____		
Time	**Urinated in Toilet**	**Amount and Type of Drink**	**Leakage** Small/Medium/Large	**Reason for Urine Leakage**	**Strong Urge?**
05:30 AM					
07:00 AM					
08:30 AM					
10:00 AM					
11:30 AM					
01:00 PM					
02:30 PM					
04:00 PM					
05:30 PM					
07:00 PM					
08:30 PM					
10:00 PM					
11:30 PM					
01:00 AM					
03:00 AM					

NOTES: _____

_____

NUMBER AND TYPE OF PADS USED TODAY: _____

_____

Bladder Diary - 1st set

Urinary Diary	Day#3		Date: _____		
Time	**Urinated in Toilet**	**Amount and Type of Drink**	**Leakage** Small/Medium/Large	**Reason for Urine Leakage**	**Strong Urge?**
05:30 AM					
07:00 AM					
08:30 AM					
10:00 AM					
11:30 AM					
01:00 PM					
02:30 PM					
04:00 PM					
05:30 PM					
07:00 PM					
08:30 PM					
10:00 PM					
11:30 PM					
01:00 AM					
03:00 AM					

NOTES: _____

_____

NUMBER AND TYPE OF PADS USED TODAY: _____

_____

Bladder Diary – 2nd set

Urinary Diary			Day#1	Date: _____	
Time	Urinated in Toilet	Amount and Type of Drink	Leakage Small/Medium/Large	Reason for Urine Leakage	Strong Urge?
05:30 AM					
07:00 AM					
08:30 AM					
10:00 AM					
11:30 AM					
01:00 PM					
02:30 PM					
04:00 PM					
05:30 PM					
07:00 PM					
08:30 PM					
10:00 PM					
11:30 PM					
01:00 AM					
03:00 AM					

NOTES: _____

_____

NUMBER AND TYPE OF PADS USED TODAY: _____

_____

Bladder Diary - 2nd set

Urinary Diary	Day#2		Date: _____		
Time	**Urinated in Toilet**	**Amount and Type of Drink**	**Leakage** Small/Medium/Large	**Reason for Urine Leakage**	**Strong Urge?**
05:30 AM					
07:00 AM					
08:30 AM					
10:00 AM					
11:30 AM					
01:00 PM					
02:30 PM					
04:00 PM					
05:30 PM					
07:00 PM					
08:30 PM					
10:00 PM					
11:30 PM					
01:00 AM					
03:00 AM					

NOTES: _____

_____

NUMBER AND TYPE OF PADS USED TODAY: _____

_____

Bladder Diary – 2nd set

Urinary Diary		Day#3	Date: _____		
Time	Urinated in Toilet	Amount and Type of Drink	Leakage Small/Medium/Large	Reason for Urine Leakage	Strong Urge?
05:30 AM					
07:00 AM					
08:30 AM					
10:00 AM					
11:30 AM					
01:00 PM					
02:30 PM					
04:00 PM					
05:30 PM					
07:00 PM					
08:30 PM					
10:00 PM					
11:30 PM					
01:00 AM					
03:00 AM					

NOTES: _____

_____

NUMBER AND TYPE OF PADS USED TODAY: _____

_____

Bladder Diary - 3rd set

Urinary Diary		Day#1		Date: _____	
Time	**Urinated in Toilet**	**Amount and Type of Drink**	**Leakage** Small/Medium/Large	**Reason for Urine Leakage**	**Strong Urge?**
05:30 AM					
07:00 AM					
08:30 AM					
10:00 AM					
11:30 AM					
01:00 PM					
02:30 PM					
04:00 PM					
05:30 PM					
07:00 PM					
08:30 PM					
10:00 PM					
11:30 PM					
01:00 AM					
03:00 AM					

NOTES: _____

_____

NUMBER AND TYPE OF PADS USED TODAY: _____

_____

Bladder Diary - 3rd set

Urinary Diary		Day#2	Date: _____		
Time	Urinated in Toilet	Amount and Type of Drink	Leakage Small/Medium/Large	Reason for Urine Leakage	Strong Urge?
05:30 AM					
07:00 AM					
08:30 AM					
10:00 AM					
11:30 AM					
01:00 PM					
02:30 PM					
04:00 PM					
05:30 PM					
07:00 PM					
08:30 PM					
10:00 PM					
11:30 PM					
01:00 AM					
03:00 AM					

NOTES: _____

_____

NUMBER AND TYPE OF PADS USED TODAY: _____

_____

Bladder Diary - 3rd set

Urinary Diary		Day#3	Date: _____		
Time	Urinated in Toilet	Amount and Type of Drink	Leakage Small/Medium/Large	Reason for Urine Leakage	Strong Urge?
05:30 AM					
07:00 AM					
08:30 AM					
10:00 AM					
11:30 AM					
01:00 PM					
02:30 PM					
04:00 PM					
05:30 PM					
07:00 PM					
08:30 PM					
10:00 PM					
11:30 PM					
01:00 AM					
03:00 AM					

NOTES: _____

_____

NUMBER AND TYPE OF PADS USED TODAY: _____

_____

Notes